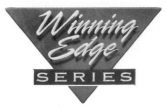

Weight Training

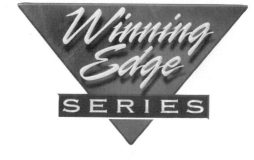

Weight Training

RICHARD W. FIELD, Ph.D.

Physical Education Instructor and Strength Coach
Albuquerque Academy

Series Editor and Co-Author
SCOTT O. ROBERTS, Ph.D.

Department of Health, Physical Education, and Recreation
Texas Tech University
Lubbock, Texas

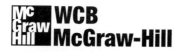

Boston   Burr Ridge, IL   Dubuque, IA   Madison, WI
New York   San Francisco   St. Louis
Bangkok   Bogotá   Caracas   Lisbon   London   Madrid   Mexico City
Milan   New Delhi   Seoul   Singapore   Sydney   Taipei   Toronto

WCB/McGraw-Hill

*A Division of The **McGraw-Hill** Companies*

WINNING EDGE SERIES: WEIGHT TRAINING

This book is printed on acid-free paper.

1 2 3 4 5 6 7 8 9 0 DOC/DOC 9 3 2 1 0 9 8

ISBN 0–8151–3324–3

Vice president and editorial director: *Kevin T. Kane*
Publisher: *Edward E. Bartell*
Executive editor: *Vicki Malinee*
Editorial coordinator: *Tricia R. Musel*
Senior marketing manager: *Pamela S. Cooper*
Editing associate: *Joyce Watters*
Production supervisor: *Deborah Donner*
Coordinator of freelance design: *Michelle D. Whitaker*
Senior photo research coordinator: *Lori Hancock*
Supplement coordinator: *David A. Welsh*
Compositor: *Shepard Poorman Communications Corp.*
Typeface: *10/12 Palatino*
Printer: *R.R Donnelley & Sons Company/Crawfordsville, IN*

Cover image: © *Bill Leslie Photography*

Coventry University

Library of Congress Cataloging-in-Publication Data

Field, Richard W.
  Weight training / Richard W. Field, Scott O. Roberts. — 1st ed.
    p. cm. — (Winning edge series)
  Includes bibliographical references (p.   ) and index.
  ISBN 0–8151–3324–3
  I.   Weight training.   2.   Physical education and training.
  I.   Roberts, Scott.   II.   Title.   III.   Series: Winning edge series
  (Boston, Mass.)
  GV546.F525   1999
  613.7'13—dc21   98–38603
                                                                CIP

www.mhhe.com

PREFACE

Welcome to the world of weight training! The purpose of this book is to help you develop strength, which will help you perform better in sports, improve your overall health, and give you positive self-esteem. Weight training can be one of the keys to improving athletic performance, rehabilitating an injury, or improving lifetime fitness.

Adequate strength is an important characteristic of good health that everyone should strive for, especially as one gets older. As a sport, weight training is accessible to all ages, gender, body types, and fitness levels. Whatever your starting point, whether you want to lose weight, "bulk up," or get stronger, there is a fitness program to help you get started. This book teaches you the basics regarding exercise selection, muscle group usage, program development, and advanced training techniques.

▶ Audience

This book is designed for anyone interested in improving his or her fitness through the popular sport of weight training. It is intended to be a manual for beginners to advanced trainees. Teachers, trainers, and coaches will also find *Weight Training* to be a useful adjunct in their respective fields.

▶ Features

The information provided in this text will allow you to use it for the rest of your life because it contains a basic lifestyle lesson of attending to your body. For anyone interested in weight training, especially beginners, this book contains great explanations, examples, and illustrations to inform you of proper techniques and ways to avoid injury. The first couple of chapters detail not only what weight lifting is all about but also present proper nutrition guidelines and training principles. Chapter 5 dedicates space to advising what program might be best for you. Thereafter, individual chapters address each muscle region and offer an array of exercises to perform.

In addition, *Weight Training* offers some special features in this book, including:

- Professional photographs to illustrate proper techniques.
- A bulleted list of objectives at the beginning of each chapter and a closing summary to outline and reinforce the major points of coverage.
- Special Fitness Tip boxes that outline concepts, applications, and procedures for quick reference.
- Appendix provides a model to develop a twelve-week complete body strength assessment program.

▶ Ancillaries

To facilitate use of this text in the classroom, a printed Test Bank of approximately 150 questions is available to instructors. These questions allow for quick assessment of the basic rules and principles of weight training. Please contact your sales representative for additional information.

▶ Acknowledgments

We would like to thank the following individuals who assisted our learning about the weight training field.

Tony Fitton

Vicki Steenrod

Larry Grier

Leo Totten

Tom Fahey

William O. Roberts

We would also like to thank New Mexico Sports and Wellness for allowing us to use the gym for photo sessions. Finally, we would like to thank the models who so graciously assisted in demonstrating the exercises shown within this text.

Shirley Roach

Roy Jennings

Alice Chung

Mitzi Lynn Keegan

—Richard W. Field

—Scott O. Roberts

CONTENTS

CHAPTER 1

LIFTING **WEIGHTS:**
WHAT'S IT ALL ABOUT?

OBJECTIVES

After reading this chapter, you should be able to do the following:

- List key benefits of weight training.
- Know the general guidelines for safe and effective weight training.
- Name several pioneers in the field of weight training.
- Understand the origins of the American and European bodybuilding and weight lifting facets of weight training.

KEY TERMS

While reading this chapter, you will become familiar with the following terms:

- ▶ Agonist
- ▶ Antagonist
- ▶ Barbell
- ▶ Bent Press
- ▶ Clean and Jerk
- ▶ Dumbbell
- ▶ Hypertrophy
- ▶ Kettlebell
- ▶ Muscle Mass
- ▶ Muscular Endurance

Continued on p. 2.

KEY TERMS

Continued from p. 1.

- ► Olympic Lifting
- ► Physical Culture
- ► Powerlifting
- ► Repetitions

- ► Sets
- ► Snatch
- ► Spotting
- ► Strength

Volenti nihil difficile. (Nothing is difficult to him who wills.)
—*Jean-Jacques Rousseau*

Welcome to the world of strength training! You don't have to be an Arnold Schwarzenneger or a Jane Fonda to appreciate the benefits of a strong, toned, and fit body. **Strength** training has developed into a high-tech, billion-dollar business. More importantly, it has become a popular way to improve athletic ability, to look and feel better, to relieve stress, and to improve overall health.

Strength training is defined as the use of different progressive resistance exercise methods designed to increase one's ability to exert muscular force against resistance. The desired outcome of strength training is obviously an improvement in strength. and sometimes includes the **hypertrophy,** or increase, of **muscle mass** as well.

Weight training typically uses common forms of equipment such as free weights or machines to provide the resistance needed to increase strength. As adaptations occur, more weight is added to provide additional resistance.

Resistance training includes the use of multiple forms of resistance when performing different exercises. Resistance can be provided by opposing muscle groups, the individual's body weight, elastic bands or tubing, and/or with free weights or machines.

The intended outcomes of resistance training include increased muscular strength and **muscular endurance**. Because resistance training is more comprehensive in scope, and because weight training usually assumes that free weights or machines are needed, the terms "resistance training" or "strength training" should be stressed over "weight training" when applied to training for health and fitness.

BENEFITS OF WEIGHT TRAINING

As we enter into the twenty-first century there is little doubt that weight training can be one of the critical contributors to an enhanced lifestyle. One study, reported in the November 1989 issue of the *Journal of the American Medical Association* found that those who exercise moderately, compared to those who do not exercise at all, reduce their risk of early death from cancer and heart disease by 50 percent! However, recent statistics indicate that only 20 percent of adults in the United States get enough regular exercise to have a positive impact on cardiovascular health; 40 percent exercise intermittently; and 40 percent are completely sedentary.

The reasons for lack of exercise may be complex, but the reasons for exercise adherence are myriad. The January 1995 issue of *Fitness Management* listed ninety-five separate health-related benefits of exercise. We will not repeat the entire list here, but some of the more pertinent benefits include: aids in weight loss, reduces risks of heart attacks and strokes, helps reduce stress, aids in controlling high blood pressure, increases bone density, boosts the immune system, reduces the risk of certain types of cancer, improves posture, and improves self-esteem. Surely there are enough reasons in this list to encourage the armchair enthusiast to become a regular participant!

The authors of this book hope that you will include weight training as part of your total fitness lifestyle and we trust that this textbook will ease your transition into becoming a lifelong weight trainer. Lifting weights will not only increase your muscular strength and endurance. By establishing a weight training program, it will also serve your fitness needs throughout your adult years.

GENERAL GUIDELINES FOR WEIGHT TRAINING

For overall safety in the weight room, the following basic rules should be observed:

1. Never lift without supervision, even if you are an experienced lifter.
2. Use collars on all free weight exercises (on both barbells and dumbbells if applicable).
3. Always have someone **spotting** on any free weight exercise where the possibility of bodily harm might be present, i.e., squats, bench (flat, incline, and decline), press behind the neck, tricep extensions, etc. NEVER attempt to spot someone doing one of the two Olympic lifts (snatch or clean and jerk), as you will endanger the lifter and yourself. Figure 1-1

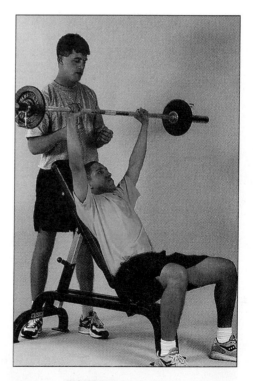

FIGURE 1-1 Spotting.

demonstrates spotting a lifter as he performs the incline press. Spotting is discussed further in chapter 6.

4. Do not attempt one-repetition maximums without competent supervision, i.e., a strength and conditioning professional. Always prepare for these test days with an adequate warm-up for each lift and plenty of rest prior to the lift. Also have alert spotters standing by to help if necessary.

5. Never deviate from proper lifting form and technique on a given exercise. Lifters (and at times spotters) are sometimes injured when attempting to squeeze out one more rep with bad form. Use proper breathing techniques: exhale on exertion, inhale when lowering the weight.

6. Always observe proper biomechanical principles when lifting. For example, lift with the legs and keep the back straight when raising a weight from the ground in a dead lift. For specifics on technique consult the technique sections of this book.

7. Lifting movements should be slow and controlled. Never hold your breath while lifting. Explosive movements would be warranted only if the athlete is training for Olympic style weight lifting.

8. Take sufficient rest periods between **sets** and **repetitions** that are appropriate to the goals you have set. Warm up prior to lifting and at each station in the routine. Get medical clearance prior to any physical conditioning program.

9. Have specific goals set for the program: strength, mass, or muscular endurance. Know your repetition and set ranges. Have a total body program with periodized cycles in place prior to beginning the lifting process.

10. Never use inappropriate behavior or dress in the weight room. The weight room is not the place for socializing, horseplay, or daydreaming. Be aware of what is going on around you at all times. Jeans, long shorts, dresses, and open-toed shoes are inappropriate for the weight room. Shorts, t-shirts, and regular activewear sneakers constitute the proper attire for working out safely.

Fitness Tip

Supportive Gear

Gloves may be worn by the beginner to help prevent blisters or to aid in gripping the barbell. Weight lifting belts are not necessary unless performing the following lifts: squats, overhead presses, bent-over rows, deadlifts, or the Olympic lifts (snatch and clean and jerk). Wraps for knees or wrists are not recommended unless the trainee has competitive aspirations in powerlifting or Olympic lifting.

TABLE 1-1
Goals and Weight Guidelines

Goal of Program	Number of Repetitions	% Intensity of 1RM*
Strength	1–10	70–100%
Muscle Mass	8–12	60–80%
Endurance	12–20	40–60%

*1RM = one repetition maximum. See chapter 4 for more information.

11. Exercise from larger and stronger muscle groups (legs, back, etc.) to smaller and weaker muscle groups (arms, abdominals). To insure balanced muscular development, always work **agonist** and **antagonist** muscles.
12. Train throughout the full range of motion.

STARTING WEIGHT

In order to start lifting, the beginning weight lifter must have an idea of the starting weight needed for each exercise. This will be determined primarily by the repetition range that you have chosen. If, for instance, you have chosen to focus on gaining mass, then an eight to twelve repetition range is appropriate. This means that if you cannot achieve at least eight repetitions with a weight, then it is too heavy. Whenever the beginner can perform twelve or more repetitions, the weight is too light and you should progress to a heavier weight.

It is also possible to choose a starting weight from a percentage chart or a repetition chart, which are commonly found in weight rooms. For example (these are only guideline weights), starting weights in the leg press should be about 100 percent of body weight, flat pulldown should be about 50 percent of body weight, the chest press about 30–50 percent, the leg curl about 30–50 percent, and the leg extension 75–100 percent of body weight. Table 1-1 provides additional guidelines for reference.

A BRIEF HISTORY OF WEIGHT LIFTING AND PHYSICAL CULTURE

▶ Professor Attila

Louis Durlacher, or Professor Attila as he was more commonly known, was born in Karlsruhe, Germany, in 1844. His early teachers in **physical culture** were Professor Ernst of Berlin and Felice Napoli of Italy. Attila trained some of the foremost leaders of physical culture and a plethora of nobles from continental Europe. Among the trainers and strength athletes trained by Attila were Sandow, Lionel

Strongfort, Rolandow, Bobby Pandour, Warren Lincoln Travis, and Professor Edmond Desbonnet (who became the father of French physical culture).

Perhaps Professor Attila's greatest contribution was the popularizing of hollow shot loading **dumbbells**. He was one of the first trainers to use cables in training and he developed the now defunct **bent press**. Attila's theories were disseminated in France by Edmond Desbonnet, in Germany by Theodor Seibert, and in the United States by Alan Calvert (who copied Seibert's program). Attila opened a physical culture studio in New York City in 1894, which would later be inherited and run by strongman son-in-law Sig Klein.

▶ Sandow

Friedrich Wilhelm Mueller (Sandow) was born in 1867 in Königsberg, East Prussia. Ostensibly the most famous of the golden age strongman performers, Sandow in his day was the embodiment of the public's perception of what a strongman should look like and the feats he should be capable of performing. In his heyday the phrase "strong as a Sandow" implied that one had reached the acme of physical perfection.

Attila met Sandow in 1887 and became his mentor in physical culture. Early in Mueller's career, Attila suggested the name change to Eugen Sandow (*Eugen* is derived from *eugenics* and *Sandow* is a Germanicized version of his mother's maiden name, Sandov). Attila encouraged the use of heavy weights in Sandow's training—against the accepted mode of training with light dumbbells—to help pack mass on the ex-circus performer.

While in Amsterdam, early in his career, Sandow used a unique stunt to drum up publicity. He went around the city covertly wrecking several coin-operated strength testing machines. These machines consisted of a lever that, when pulled downward, gave a strength rating. Sandow simply pulled the lever beyond its maximum and thereby made the machines inoperable. When arrested by the police, the authorities were stunned to find out that this vandal had been working alone; they thought that it would take the strength of several men to inflict such damage. Only when Sandow lifted the largest constable there off the floor did they believe him.

Perhaps the most famous episode in Sandow's career took place at the Royal Aquarium Music Hall in Westminster on October 29, 1889. Here two strongmen with the stage names of Sampson and Cyclops staged a nightly challenge to the audience to duplicate their feats of strength. On this evening Sandow came on stage dressed in an evening suit and monocle. He then discarded his accoutrements and lifted the challenge dumbbells and **barbells** of Cyclops. Sampson delayed his meeting with Sandow until November 2, 1889, when Sandow bent the bars, tore the wire rope, and broke the chains of Sampson. Needless to say he won the match, but failed to collect all of the promised prize money.

Sandow then started his own stage show and toured Europe, the United States, Australia, and India over a period of years. He became the first man in history to press 250 lbs. overhead and to bent press 300 lbs. His most lasting legacy, however, may have been his knack for promoting the fitness field. He published several books on strength training, opened his own physical culture schools, sold mail-order courses and exercise equipment, and crusaded for physical fitness in his adopted home, Great Britain. His physique remains with us to this day, as Sandow was the model for the original statuette created by William Pomeroy as the ultimate prize in the Mr. Olympia contests.

▶ Apollon

Louis Uni was born in 1862 in Marsillargues, France, and went by the stage name of Apollon. Apollon stood 6' 2.8" tall and weighed 260 lbs. at his most muscular condition. He was most widely recognized for his grip and forearm strength.

One of his greatest feats took place during a regular stage performance. During his act he would portray a prisoner trying to escape from his guards and would force apart iron bars. However, before a performance in 1889, someone had bribed the blacksmith who restraightened his bars to temper or harden them. When confronted with these bars, Apollon was at first unable to bend them until goaded into action by his petite wife who waited in the wings. Summoning all of his strength in a genuine effort, he finally forced his way through and was so exhausted that he had to conclude his act for the night.

On another occasion, Apollon was performing at the Varieties Theatre in Lille in 1892. A rival group of strongmen, three Germans known as the Rasso Trio, were in town to catch his act and if possible usurp his title of "Strongest Man." With this knowledge, Apollon asked his friend and fellow strongman Batta to upgrade the weight in one of his barbells so that it would weigh more (by adding sand in the hollow spheres). While changing the weight Batta was approached by the wrestler Paul Pons, who suggested adding iron spheres instead of sand, raising the barbell's weight from 198 lbs. to 341 lbs. (in addition this barbell had a thick 2.5" handle). Apollon began his performance with several feats using lighter bells. Then came the moment of truth as the thick-handled barbell was rolled out. Yet the French strongman never waivered, **clean and jerking** the huge weight overhead with ease. He finished the feat by holding the bar aloft with one hand while raising his right leg straight out to his side!

His most legendary feat was the overhead lifting of the "wheels of Apollon," a pair of railway wheels mounted on an axle, which weighed 367 lbs. Only such luminaries as Rigolout and John Davis could equal this feat.

▶ Arthur Saxon

Arthur Hennig Saxon was born in 1878 in Leipzig, Germany. He was the central figure in the group of strongmen known as the Arthur Saxon Trio, which operated between the years of 1897 and 1914. This trio contained various other strongmen (such as Adolf Berg) until Arthur's brothers Hermann and Kurt were mature enough to join the act.

The brothers first practiced lifting stone weights and **kettlebells** in their parents' home (see Figure 1-2 for an example of these weights). At age 16, Arthur joined the Atlas club in Leipzig and was acknowledged as the strongest man in the club shortly thereafter. Arthur became a specialist in the one-handed lifts, in particular the bent

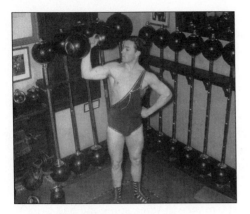

FIGURE 1-2 Kettlebells.

press, in which his official record consisted of a staggering 335.75 lbs. This lift, which is no longer practiced, was performed at the South London Palace on January 4, 1905.

The following were his best lifts at a body weight of 190–200 lbs.: right-hand snatch, 195 lbs.; right-hand swing with dumbbell, 187 lbs.; two hands clean and jerk, 336 lbs.; two dumbbells clean and jerk, 288.5 lbs.; and barbell jerk from behind the neck, 386 lbs.

The trio disbanded due to World War I and Arthur Saxon died in Duisburg, Germany, in 1921 at age 43.

▶ Katie Sandwina

Austrian strongwoman Katie Brumbach (Sandwina was a stage name patterned after Sandow) stood 5'11" and weighed 209.5 lbs. Although not much is known of her early life, she was the daughter of Philip Brumbach, a strongman finger-lifting champion. A pioneer in the field of women's lifting and stage performance strongwoman acts, Sandwina was also a star attraction in Barnum and Bailey's Circus from 1911 to 1912. Her best lifts were shouldering and then jerking 264.55 lbs. and a one-arm jerk of 176.36 lbs. Her feats were not to be equaled or surpassed until the second half of the twentieth century.

▶ Henry "Milo" Steinborn

Born in 1894, Milo Steinborn came to the United States in 1921, shortly after his internment in a prisoner of war camp in New South Wales (he had fought on the German side during World War I). He almost single-handedly made the squat a popular exercise in the United States. He was prominently featured in *Strength* magazine and Alan Calvert's book, *Super-Strength*. In addition, another great squatter, Sig Klein, regularly dispensed stories of Steinborn's squatting prowess to eager fans of the iron game.

In New York, in 1921, he squatted with 550 lbs. at a body weight of 210 lbs. He also once squatted with 315 lbs. thirty-three times successively, and did a one-leg squat with 192 lbs. Steinborn was also very strong in other lifts: 353.5 lbs. in the two-arm clean and jerk; a one-arm snatch of 208 lbs.; and two-handed military press, 265 lbs.

Milo continued a career as a professional wrestler long after his glory days as a lifter had passed. A picture taken of him in 1955 (when he was sixty-one) with his twenty-two-year-old son, Henry Jr., shows that he retained much of his powerful physique in his later years.

► Louis Cyr

Louis Cyr was born in 1863 in the small village of St. Cyprien de Naperville, near Montreal, Canada. Fully grown, he stood 5' 8.5" tall and weighed between 270 and 315 lbs. He showed his strength early on when, at the age of seventeen, he used a back lift to raise up a wagon stuck in the mud until the driver's horses pulled it out of the muck. At eighteen, he was matched in a boulder lifting contest against the strongest man in Canada, David Michaud. Cyr out lifted Michaud by raising a granite boulder weighing 480 lbs.

After a short stint as a lumberjack, Cyr began training with weights in preparation for a career as a strongman. One of Cyr's most celebrated incidents involved his subduing two knife fighting punks while working as a patrolman outside of Montreal. Not only did he subdue them, but he then proceeded to carry them back to his station, one under each arm! Shortly after this, sports promoter Richard Fox backed Cyr as the "Strongest Man in the World" and offered $5,000 to anyone who could duplicate Cyr's feats of strength. Cyr defeated many famous strongmen, but Sandow, who was in his prime at the time, ignored Cyr's repeated challenges to a championship match.

Cyr's most famous lift was the back lift in which he claimed a best of 4,300 lbs. In actuality, however, his best confirmed lift was 3,626 lbs. (a platform plus the weight of sixteen men)—an example of the gross exaggeration often used by strongmen in promoting their feats.

Cyr was never defeated during his long practiced (1881–1906) profession as a strongman, but he died at the young age of forty-nine in 1912.

► John Grimek

John Carl Grimek was of Czechoslovakian descent and was inspired indirectly in his early training by Earle Liedermann. His older brother had been training on a chest expander course sold by Liedermann and the younger Grimek soon caught on and was bitten by the "iron bug." In addition to his expander training, Grimek's early training consisted of kettlebell exercises, chins, and push-ups. Grimek's enthusiasm for lifting grew (and his brother moved, leaving behind all of his lifting gear) and he added some hand balancing, wrestling, and jumping to his expanding versatility.

Grimek was to become a link between the physical culturists of the "older era"—the Kleins, Hackenschmidts, Steinborns, etc.—and the newer generation of muscle stars like Steve Reeves, Reg Park, and Tommy Kono. He influenced not only the pure strength athletes, but physiquemen of his day as well. He was a world-class competitor in **Olympic lifting** for almost two decades and, at age 40, beat Steve Reeves in a Mr. Universe contest.

His best lifts include pressing a 125 lb. and a 110 lb. dumbbell simultaneously; a 258.5 lb. press; a 220 lb. **snatch;** and a 308 lb. clean and jerk (the latter three marks all coming at the Senior National Championships of 1936). Perhaps most remarkable about Grimek was his ageless physique. At age 39 his statistics were: weight, 203 lbs.; chest, 50"; neck, 17.75"; waist, 30.5"; arm, 18.5"; thigh, 25.75"; and calf

17.25". Of John Grimek's lasting legacy to the field physical culture it may truly be said that he is *"sui generis,"* or "one of a kind."

▶ John Davis

John Davis was born in 1921 in Smithtown, Long Island, New York. In his early years, Davis excelled in handball, swimming, running, jumping, and assorted strength feats. Although an Olympic lifting specialist, he recorded a 700 lb. dead-lift, squatted 525 lbs. eight times, two-arm curled 215 lbs., clean and jerked two 142 lb. dumbbells, and bench pressed 425 lbs.

It was in Olympic lifting, however, that Davis was to leave his greatest efforts. He was undefeated as a heavyweight lifter from 1938 until 1953. Davis also held all records—national, world, and Olympic—at the same time in his stellar career. He was the first man to jerk 400 lbs. and his all-time best lifts were: press, 342 lbs.; snatch, 330.5 lbs.; and the clean and jerk, 402 lbs. And lest anyone forget, he clean and jerked the Apollon railway wheels on September 13, 1949.

Davis was a great lifting talent and certainly one of the all-time greats in American and international weight lifting circles. He was also a role model for young African Americans, for although he was not the first African American in weight lifting, his supremacy in his field of endeavor brought him the respect and admiration of people from around the world and helped to break down barriers of race and color.

▶ Doug Hepburn

Douglas Hepburn was born in Vancouver, British Columbia, in 1927. He went on to become a "giant" of weight lifting in stature as well as accomplishments despite a club foot on the right side, which was later operated on, causing some bones in the right ankle to fuse together. At his peak, Hepburn stood 5'8" and weighed 250 lbs., although he sometimes ranged as high as 280 to 300 lbs. in body weight. His best lifts were: two hands press off the rack, 440 lbs.; two hands press with dumbbells, 350 lbs. (175 lbs. each); press behind the neck, 350 lbs.; two hands curl, 260 lbs.; bench press, 580 lbs.; jerk-press off the rack, 500 lbs., two hands snatch, 297.5 lbs.; two hands clean and press, 381 lbs.; squat, 760 lbs.; two hands deadlift, 705 lbs.; two hands dumbbell jerk, 314 lbs. (154 lbs. each).

Eventually, even the great John Davis, who had reigned for fifteen years as the undefeated heavyweight champion, succumbed to Doug Hepburn. In 1953, in Stockholm, Sweden, Hepburn totaled 1,030.5 lbs. (the highest total ever made up to that point) in the three Olympic lifts to beat Davis by 22.25 lbs. Perhaps it was no exaggeration when Joe Weider said of Hepburn: "One of these days, the full story of Hepburn will be told and when it is it will serve forever as an inspiration to us all—for it will tell how a boy overcame a physical handicap to become the GREATEST OF THEM ALL."

▶ Tommy Kono

Tommy Kono was born in 1930. When he was just eleven years old, weighing only 74.5 lbs. and standing 4' 8.5" tall, Kono answered a Charles Atlas ad, but was unable to afford the course. During World War II, Kono and his family (of Japanese American origin) were interned for three and a half years at Tule Lake, California. It was during this stay that a teacher introduced Kono to weight training. At age 16, Kono began Olympic lifting at the Sacramento YMCA. He joined Ed Yarick's gym, where he received great motivational support, in 1949.

Kono went on to become America's greatest Olympic lifter, winning three Olympic medals. He won two gold medals in 1952 and 1956 and one silver medal in 1960. Although he competed in the 67.5 kilo (148.5 lbs.), 75.0 kilo (165 lbs.), and 82.5 kilo (181.5 lbs.) classes, his best lifts were in the latter two classes. In the 75.0 kilo class he had a 145.5 kilo (320.1 lbs.) press, a 133.5 kilo (293.7 lbs.) snatch, a 176.0 kilo (387.2 lbs.) clean and jerk, and a 430.0 kilo (946 lbs.) total. In the 82.5 kilo class he performed a World Record 153.0 kilo (336.6 lbs.) press, a 137.5 kilo (302.5 lbs.) snatch, a 170.0 kilo (374 lbs.) clean and jerk, and a World Record 460.0 kilo (1012 lbs.) total in the Prize of Moscow Tournament in March of 1961.

In a 1982 poll conducted by the World Weight Lifting Federation, Tommy Kono was voted the greatest weight lifter of all time by a worldwide panel of journalists and sports writers. He continues to inspire new generations of lifters.

▶ Eddie Ignacious Coan

Eddie Coan was born in 1963 and first became interested in lifting when, as an eighth grader, he watched the film *Pumping Iron*. He then began training in a friend's basement and joined the wrestling team. Although a diminutive 4'11" and 98 lbs. when he started, Coan continued to train and grow in size and strength. In 1980 he watched Bill Kazmaier compete on TV and decided to gain weight and compete himself. In his first **powerlifting** meet at a body weight of 165 lbs., he squatted 485 lbs., benched 295 lbs., and deadlifted 495 lbs.

Coan is presently 5'6" tall and weighs 220 lbs. He is the eight-time World Champion, two-time YMCA National Champion, 1985 Hawaiian Invitational Champion, eleven-time Senior Nationals Champion, and is currently recognized as the strongest male powerlifter in the world today.

He currently holds the following records in the 181 lb. class: deadlift, 793 lbs.; squat, 859 lbs.; deadlift, 859 lbs.; total 2,204 lbs. in the 198 lb. class; squat, 964 lbs.; deadlift, 901 lbs.; total 2,402 lbs. in the 220 lb. class. He also boasts a best bench of 562 lbs. and can do 500 lbs. for five reps (no wraps) on his favorite exercise, the bent-over row on a 3" block. Coan is simply "in a class by himself."

▶ Vicki Steenrod

Vicki Steenrod was born in 1949 in Freeport, Illinois, the oldest daughter of Joyce and Vito Di Modica. Vicki began lifting weights in 1979 while a student at the University of New Mexico. She was encouraged at this stage by Pete Martinelli, the UNM strength coach, who was one of the few proponents of weight training for women at that time. Vicki entered her first Nationals in 1981 and won her first Nationals in 1982. Since then, she has won nine more National titles (see Figure 1-3). She is the only woman to have won ten National titles in powerlifting (only two men have achieved the same level of excellence).

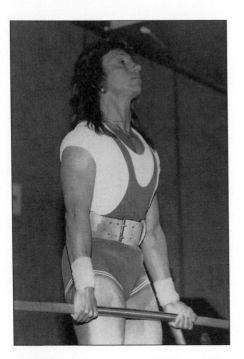

FIGURE 1-3 Vicki Steenrod at the 1983 Chicago Nationals.

In 1984, Vicki became the first woman to bench press double her body weight with an official lift of 248 lbs. while weighing 123 lbs. This was an official world record and in the eleven years following this landmark lift, the world record for this class has only been surpassed by a five-pound margin. Also in 1984, Vicki (along with another woman) made the qualifying total for the men's Nationals (up to this time only men had competed in this division, as no one expected a female to total that amount). It was the first and last time such an "affront" to the male domain was allowed. In 1985, the Nationals was renamed the Men's Nationals.

Vicki Steenrod has broken many U.S. and world records during her career. At present, Vicki still holds two world records, one in the 132 lb. class (set in 1985) and the other in the 148 lb. class. Since turning forty years of age, Vicki has been entitled to compete in the Master division in which she won the world title in 1993 and established all the world records in the 165 lb. class. She had previously won four open world titles: 1984, 1985, 1987, and 1989.

When Vicki started competing in 1980, she weighed 114 lbs., now she weighs around 170 lbs. During these fifteen years, Vicki has established all the New Mexico state records in five different weight classes, and has held U.S. and world records in four different weight classes. Vicki Steenrod's best lifts at a body weight of 165 pounds are: squat, 480 lbs.; bench press, 330 lbs.; and deadlift, 485 lbs.

SUMMARY

- Some of the important benefits of weight training and exercise include: weight loss and weight control, reduction in stress levels, improved posture, improved self-esteem, increased strength and muscular endurance, and reduced risk of heart attack and stroke.
- Never lift without supervision AND proper instruction.
- Always use spotters on free weight exercises like the squat, bench press, or any overhead lift. Use correct form and follow basic biomechanical principles.

- Lifters should always start a program with a specific goal in mind: i.e., mass, strength, or muscular endurance. Lifting should always be slow and controlled. Avoid lifting heavy weight simply to impress your friends.
- Modern-day bodybuilding has its origins in the physical culturists of the latter part of the nineteenth century. Olympic lifting is the oldest competitive form of weight lifting. Powerlifting is a relatively recent addition (1960s).

▶ **Agonist   p. 5**
The prime mover or major muscle involved in an exercise.

▶ **Antagonist   p. 5**
The major muscle that relaxes in response to the prime mover in an exercise.

▶ **Barbell   p. 6**
A long bar (usually 7 feet in length) weighing forty-five pounds. Additional weights may be added to the ends of the bar in the form of weight plates.

▶ **Bent Press   p. 6**
A lift that is no longer contested. This lift began with the bar on the lifter's shoulder. He would then press the bar away from his body as his torso went into a position parallel with the floor.

▶ **Clean and Jerk   p. 7**
This is one of the two Olympic lifts. In this movement the athlete first lifts (cleans) the weight to his chest and then, while splitting his stance, jerks it overhead.

▶ **Dumbbell   p. 6**
A small weight (usually ranging from 5 to 100 pounds) that is held with one hand. It may be used alone or one may be used in each hand to complete an exercise.

▶ **Hypertrophy   p. 2**
Increase in muscle fiber size due to training.

▶ **Kettlebell   p. 7**
An older type of weight, rarely seen today, that was globe-shaped with a fixed handle. It was generally used for dumbbell-type exercises.

▶ **Muscle Mass   p. 2**
The parts of the body composed of lean muscle tissue.

▶ **Muscular Endurance   p.2**
The ability of a muscle or muscle group to exert force repeatedly against a resistance.

▶ **Olympic Lifting   p. 9**
The two overhead weight lifts (the snatch and the clean and jerk) contested at the Olympic games (the press was dropped in the 1970s). Three attempts are given on each of the two lifts and the best lift in each goes toward a combined total.

▶ **Physical Culture   p. 5**
The term for bodybuilding and weight training in the late nineteenth and early twentieth centuries.

▶ **Powerlifting   p. 11**
This weight lifting sport consists of three lifts contested in this order: squat, bench press, and deadlift. The best lifts from all three categories are added up for the combined total.

▶ **Repetitions   p. 4**

Each time the weight is moved up and down counts as one repetition. Repetitions should be slow and controlled.

▶ **Sets   p. 4**

A group of repetitions. For example, one set might equal twelve repetitions.

▶ **Snatch   p. 9**

The first Olympic lift in a contest. In this movement the athlete pulls the bar from the floor to the overhead position in one explosive, continuous motion.

▶ **Spotting   p. 3**

When an assistant stands by and aids if necessary in the performance of a potentially difficult lift.

▶ **Strength   p. 2**

The ability to exert muscular force against resistance.

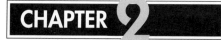

CHAPTER 2

YOUR BODY AND
WEIGHT LIFTING

OBJECTIVES

After reading this chapter, you should be able to do the following:

- Define muscular strength and endurance.
- Explain the difference between an isometric, isotonic and isokinetic contraction.
- Describe the difference between variable resistance and isokinetic exercise equipment.
- Understand how muscles get larger and stronger.

KEY TERMS

While reading this chapter, you will become familiar with the following terms:

- ► Concentric Muscle Contractions
- ► Eccentric Muscle Contractions
- ► Fast Twitch Fiber
- ► Isokinetic Movement

- ► Isometric Contraction
- ► Isotonic Contraction
- ► Motor Unit
- ► Muscle Fibers

Continued on p. 16.

Continued from p. 15.

KEY TERMS

- Muscular Endurance
- Muscular Hypertrophy
- Muscular Strength
- Negative Exercises

- Slow Twitch Fiber
- Sticking Point
- Variable or Accommodating Resistance Equipment

PHYSIOLOGICAL EFFECTS OF STRENGTH TRAINING

MUSCLE

Muscles are comprised of bundles of individual muscle fibers bound together by specialized connective tissue. If you were to take a look at a cross-section view of human skeletal muscle, it would have the appearance of a telephone or television cord containing hundreds of small wires bound together. Individual **muscle fibers** are the smallest division of muscle. These fibers are very small, and can only be seen under a microscope. There are three primary muscle fibers: **fast twitch** (IIb fibers), intermediate (IIa fibers) and **slow twitch** (I fibers).

The composition of the fibers in your body is primarily genetically predetermined. Slow twitch fibers are highly aerobic, richly supplied with blood, slow to fatigue, and contract slowly. Fast twitch fibers have the opposite properties (highly anaerobic, poor blood supply, fast to fatigue, and contract fast).World-class runners have 60 to 90 percent slow twitch fibers, whereas world-class weight lifters have 60 to 70 percent fast twitch fibers. The average sedentary individual has 40 to 50 percent slow twitch fibers and the rest a combination of fast twitch and intermediate fibers.

Each skeletal muscle fiber is connected to a nerve fiber called a motor neuron, which extends outward from the spinal column. The motor neuron and the muscle fibers it is connected to is called a **motor unit**.

HOW MUSCLES GET BIGGER AND STRONGER

Improvements in strength are initially related to neural adaptations. When a muscle is stimulated to contract, one or many motor units may be stimulated to contract. The greater the number of motor units stimulated, the greater the strength of contraction, and thus the more weight that can be lifted. When motor units are recruited in selected patterns, individuals are able to lift more weight. Strength training improves the nervous system's ability to coordinate the recruitment of muscle fibers.

Later, muscle cells actually increase in size, which is referred to as **muscular hypertrophy**. The greater the cross-sectional area of muscle, the greater force that can be generated. Larger muscles are stronger muscles. The reason bodybuilders' muscles are so large is because the individual muscle fibers have increased in size over time as a direct result of training. Thus, improvements in muscular strength and size are due to improved neural adaptations and muscular hypertrophy (see Figure 2-1).

GENDER DIFFERENCES IN STRENGTH DEVELOPMENT

Both men and women should be encouraged to get involved in a strength and weight training program. Women can gain significant levels of strength from training. Girls and boys appear to have similar levels of strength before puberty. After puberty, boys are able to develop greater levels of strength, primarily because of increased amounts of the male hormone testosterone. The benefits of strength and weight training are the same for both sexes. Today, women of all ages are participating in strength and weight training programs with terrific results.

Women are often concerned that they will get "really big" muscles from strength training. Actually, it is physiologically impossible for women to develop "huge" muscles, like those seen on male bodybuilders. It is true that women's muscles will be slightly larger and more defined after strength training. However, strength training is a great way for women to get in shape and provides numerous health benefits.

DEFINING MUSCULAR STRENGTH AND MUSCULAR ENDURANCE

Adequate strength and flexibility are important components of health- and performance-related fitness, and overall good health and well-being. Poor muscular strength and flexibility can lead to serious health problems. The majority of chronic low back pain is due to a loss in muscle mass and flexibility. A decline in lean body mass, usually as a result of physical inactivity, is associated with a decrease in basal metabolic rate (BMR), which usually leads to an increase in body fat.

Adequate **muscular strength** and **muscular endurance** are also important to success in different sports. Thus, muscular strength and flexibility should be assessed on a regular basis as part of a comprehensive health and/or fitness screening, and to help develop and analyze physical fitness and sport training programs.

An **isotonic contraction** (*iso*—equal, and *tonic*—tension) is a dynamic contraction in which the muscles generate force against a constant resistance, but not constant force or tension (example, free weights). During an isotonic movement, the force or tension required to lift a weight through a given range of motion will vary

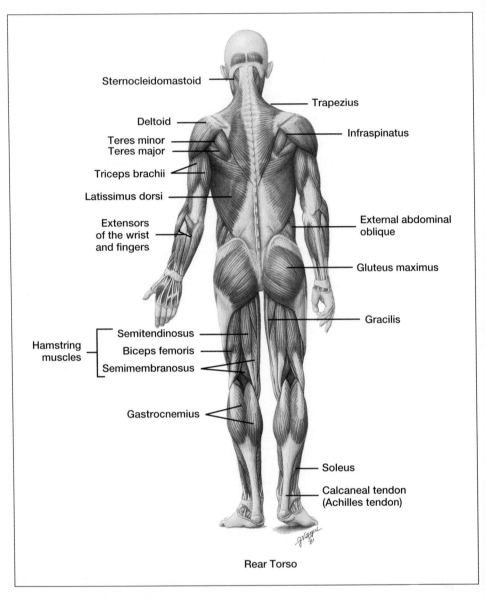

FIGURE 2-1A Major muscles of the body.

according to the joint angle. For example, when performing a bicep curl with a 50 lb. dumbbell, the tension or force (force = F) required to lift the weight is 50 lbs. at the start of the movement 0° (arm straight down), is greatest at 90° (F = 65 lbs.) (forearm parallel to the floor), and is lowest at 180° (F = 32.5 lbs.) (fully contracted toward your chest).

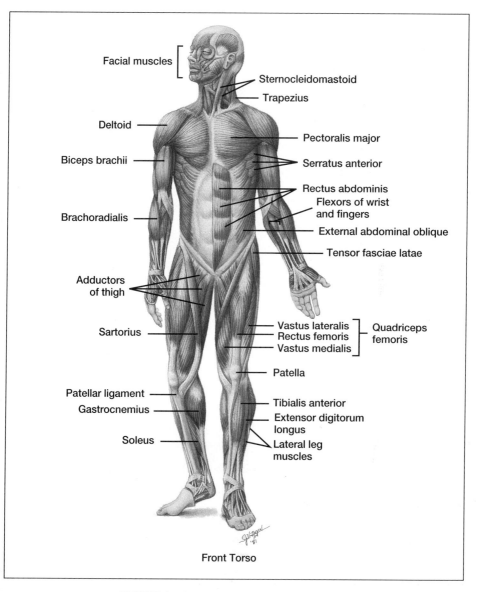

Facial muscles
Sternocleidomastoid
Trapezius
Deltoid
Pectoralis major
Biceps brachii
Serratus anterior
Rectus abdominis
Flexors of wrist and fingers
Brachoradialis
External abdominal oblique
Tensor fasciae latae
Adductors of thigh
Sartorius
Vastus lateralis
Rectus femoris
Vastus medialis
Quadriceps femoris
Patella
Patellar ligament
Gastrocnemius
Tibialis anterior
Extensor digitorum longus
Soleus
Lateral leg muscles

Front Torso

FIGURE 2-1B Major muscles of the body.

Isotonic movements consist of **concentric** and **eccentric** muscle contractions. The concentric phase of an isotonic muscular contraction occurs when the muscles contract and shorten, as when you are lifting a weight up toward your chest during a bicep curl. The eccentric phase of an isotonic contraction occurs when the muscles relax and lengthen, as when releasing the weight down during a bicep curl. Figure 2-2 illustrates both types of contractions.

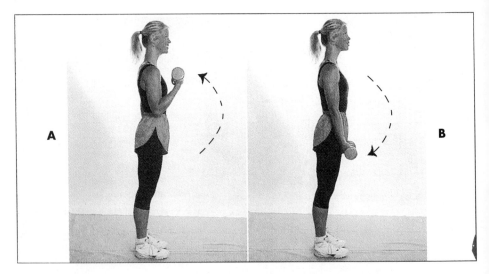

FIGURE 2-2 **A.** A concentric contraction. **B.** An eccentric contraction.

Fitness Tip

The Sticking Point

The force required to lift a set amount of weight during an isotonic movement is not constant throughout the full range of motion, meaning that there is an easy point in the lift and a hard point. In weight lifting circles the hardest part of the lift is referred to as the **sticking point**. This point in the lift is harder because your muscles are weakest at this point in the movement. When performing the bicep curl, the hardest part in the lift is at approximately 90° to 100°, or when your forearm is parallel to the floor. Even though you may be able to lift a 50 lb. dumbbell at the start of the movement from 0° to 80° and at the end of the lift from 100° to 180°, you may not be able to lift it through the "sticking point" from 90° to 100°. If you are having trouble moving a given amount of weight past a sticking point in a particular exercise, try the following: (1) perform the exercise using accommodating resistance exercises, (2) use isometric exercises at the sticking point to build up additional strength specific to that joint angle, or (3) perform "negatives" through the sticking point (see next tip box).

Fitness Tip

Negative Exercises

Exercises that rely mainly on eccentric movements are referred to as **negative exercises** or eccentric training. Negative exercises are commonly performed with the use of a partner. For example, in a negative bicep curl the assisting partner lifts a barbell up into position, 180° of the bicep curl, and then the lifter slowly lets the weight back down to 0°. The amount of the weight lifted is typically more than the lifter could lift alone. This first example is a completely eccentric movement. For the next repetition, the assisting partner may pick the weight up and move it back into position or assist the lifter with the concentric phase of the movement. Eccentric training has been shown to produce greater strength gains than strictly concentric and eccentric training together. However, eccentric training produces greater fatigue and increases the risk of injury significantly.

An **isometric contraction** is a static contraction in which the muscle generates force against an immovable object with no muscle shortening taking place. Attempting to lift or push an immovable object (a car with its brakes on) is an example of an isometric contraction. Isometric exercises can produce significant strength gains, but only at the angle at which the isometric contraction is performed.

VARIABLE RESISTANCE EQUIPMENT

During an isotonic movement (e.g., the bicep curl), the amount of force needed to move the weight from start to finish (180° movement) changes according to the joint angle. Once the inertia of the weight has been overcome and momentum has been established, the force needed to lift the weight is greatest at approximately 90°(the midpoint of the movement) and the least at approximately 180°(the finishing point). Thus, during an isotonic movement, the weight is constant, but the muscular force needed to move the weight varies.

The disadvantage of isotonic testing and training equipment is that the resistance is always changing throughout the range of motion. In an effort to create a more constant resistance during exercise movements, companies have developed **variable** or **accommodating resistance** equipment, such as Nautilus and Universal equipment. Nautilus equipment uses specially shaped devices (kidney shaped cams) to alter the resistance throughout the range of motion, whereas Universal equipment uses a special design to achieve the same results. By using varying or accommodating equipment, the force needed to move weight is increased at the joint angle and muscle length that is mechanically advantaged (180° during the bicep curl) and decreased at the joint angle that is mechanically disadvantaged (90° during the bicep curl).

ISOKINETIC EQUIPMENT

An **isokinetic movement** is one in which the length of the muscle changes while the contraction is performed at a constant velocity. During an isotonic movement, the velocity of the movement is not always constant. With isokinetic devices, however, the resistance is constant and maximum throughout the full range of motion. No matter how much force is applied, the speed of the movement is always the same. With isokinetic equipment, peak power or force can be achieved throughout the full range of motion. A variety of isokinetic devices are available today (Cybex, Biodex, Lido, KinCom).

SUMMARY

- Muscles are comprised of bundles of individual muscle fibers bound together by specialized connective tissue. There are three primary muscle fibers: fast twitch (IIb fibers), intermediate (IIa fibers), and slow twitch (I fibers).
- Improvements in strength are initially related to neural adaptations. Later, muscle cells actually increase in size, which is referred to as muscular hypertrophy.
- The benefits of strength and weight training are the same for both sexes.
- Adequate strength and flexibility are important components of health- and performance-related fitness, and overall good health and well-being.
- Muscular strength is defined as the greatest amount of force a muscle or group of muscles can produce during one maximal isotonic, isometric, or isokinetic contraction. Muscular endurance is the ability of a muscle or muscle group to perform repeated contractions for an extended period of time.
- There are three types of muscular contraction: isotonic (comprised of concentric and eccentric movements), isometric, and isokinetic.
- The sticking point is the hardest part of an isotonic movement.
- Eccentric training has been shown to produce greater strength gains than strictly concentric and eccentric training together. However, eccentric training produces greater fatigue and increases the risk of injury significantly.
- Varying or accommodating equipment increases the force needed to move weight at the joint angle and muscle length that is mechanically advantaged (180° during the bicep curl) and decreases the force needed at the joint angle that is mechanically disadvantaged (90° during the bicep curl). With isokinetic devices, the resistance is constant and maximum throughout the full range of motion. No matter how much force is applied, the speed of the movement is always the same.

▶ **Concentric Muscle Contractions**   **p. 19**
The concentric phase of an isotonic muscular contraction occurs when the muscles contract and shorten.

▶ **Eccentric Muscle Contractions**   **p. 19**
The eccentric phase of an isotonic muscular contraction occurs when the muscles relax and lengthen.

▶ **Fast Twitch Fiber (type IIb fibers)**   **p. 16**
These muscle fibers are highly anaerobic, receive a poor blood supply, fatigue quickly, and contract fast.

▶ **Isokinetic Movement**   **p. 22**
A movement in which the length of the muscle changes while the contraction is performed at a constant velocity.

▶ **Isometric Contraction**   **p. 21**
A static contraction in which the muscle generates force against an immovable object with no muscle shortening taking place.

▶ **Isotonic Contraction (*iso*—equal, and *tonic*—tension)**   **p. 17**
A dynamic contraction in which the muscles generate force against a constant resistance, but not constant force or tension (example, free weights).

▶ **Motor Unit**   **p. 16**
The motor neuron and the muscle fibers it is connected to.

▶ **Muscle Fibers**   **p. 16**
The smallest division of muscle.

▶ **Muscular Endurance**   **p. 17**
The ability of a muscle or muscle group to perform repeated contractions for an extended period of time.

▶ **Muscular Hypertrophy**   **p. 17**
The increase in cross-sectional area of muscle following strength training.

▶ **Muscular Strength**   **p. 17**
The greatest amount of force a muscle or group of muscles can produce during one maximal contraction.

▶ **Negative Exercises**   **p. 21**
Exercises that rely mainly on eccentric movements.

▶ **Slow Twitch Fiber (type I fibers)**   **p. 16**
These muscle fibers are highly aerobic, richly supplied with blood, slow to fatigue, and contract slowly.

▶ **Sticking Point**   **p. 20**
The hardest part of an isotonic movement.

▶ **Variable or Accommodating Resistance Equipment**   **p. 21**
Specialized exercise equipment that alters the force needed to overcome the resistance throughout the range of motion of selected exercises.

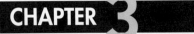
PROPER NUTRITION:
KEY TO SUCCESS

OBJECTIVES

After reading this chapter, you should be able to do the following:

- List the six basic categories of nutrition.
- Know what comprises a health-supporting diet.
- Indicate the protein requirements for active individuals.
- Understand how to use the Food Guide Pyramid.
- Explain the importance of good nutrition for athletic performance.

KEY TERMS

While reading this chapter, you will become familiar with the following terms:

- ► Carbohydrates
- ► Essential Amino Acids
- ► Fats
- ► Food Guide Pyramid
- ► Minerals
- ► Nitrogen Balance
- ► Nonessential Amino Acids
- ► Nutrient Density
- ► Protein
- ► Vitamins

BASIC NUTRITION PRINCIPLES

Proper nutrition is important to anyone involved in a serious strength or endurance training program. Just pick up any fitness magazine today and you will be inundated with advertisements for nutrition supplements promoting everything from improved strength to increased longevity. However, you should not be fooled by the majority of these claims. Although most nutrition supplements will not harm you (unless taken in large quantities), most often they do not live up to their claims. The majority of medical and nutrition experts agree that everyone, including athletes, should obtain their individual nutritional requirements through eating the right foods, and not through nutrition supplements. Once you learn how to eat a balanced diet, you should be able to get all of your daily nutrition requirements from the foods you eat.

There are approximately fifty nutrients in food that are believed to be essential for the body's growth, maintenance, and repair. These are classified into six categories: carbohydrates, fats, protein, vitamins, minerals, and water. The first three provide energy, which is measured in calories. All six are important for normal bodily functions. A health-supporting diet should be composed of 50 to 60 percent carbohydrates, 25 to 30 percent fat, and 10 to 15 percent protein. The best way to achieve a balanced diet is to eat a variety of foods, and from a variety of food groups. The Food Guide Pyramid (discussed later in this chapter) has been developed to help you make the right nutritional choices.

CARBOHYDRATES

Carbohydrates are often referred to as the body's primary fuel source because the brain burns exclusively carbohydrates, which are needed for efficient burning of fat. Carbohydrates are found almost exclusively in food from plant sources. The word *carbohydrate* comes from its chemical structure: carbon (C), hydrogen (H), and oxygen (O); thus it is abbreviated CHO.

Carbohydrates are classified as simple or complex. Examples of simple carbohydrates include table sugar, glucose, fructose, honey, and molasses. Examples of complex carbohydrates include grains, beans, potatoes, vegetables, and rice. Starches such as rice, potatoes, cereal grains, and vegetables supply not only energy, but also vitamins, minerals, fiber, and water. A healthy diet should be high in complex carbohydrates and low in simple carbohydrates. At least 50 to 60 percent of a health-supporting diet should come from complex carbohydrates. Excess consumption of simple carbohydrates can more readily be part of overeating than a diet high in complex carbohydrates. It's important to remember that following the Food Guide Pyramid and eating foods high in complex carbohydrates is usually not fattening. Carbohydrates supply only four calories per gram consumed, as compared to fats that offer nine calories per gram. Consumption of calories beyond energy use results in increased body fat.

PROTEIN

Protein is often referred to as the building block of the body because muscles are high in protein. Protein makes up approximately 18 to 20 percent of the human body. Protein is made up of compounds known as amino acids. Amino acids are joined in unique chains to form specific proteins. When protein is consumed it is broken down into amino acids during the digestive process. There are twenty common amino acids—nine **essential amino acids** and eleven **nonessential amino acids.** All amino acids are vital to human life. Essential amino acids need to be consumed in the diet because the body does not manufacture them, whereas nonessential amino acids can be synthesized by the body.

The main function of protein is growth and repair. It is the structural foundation for all body tissues. In some cases protein can also be used for energy. When protein is used for energy, it can supply four calories per gram. Proteins in food are

Fitness Tip

Vegetarian Diets

There are a variety of vegetarian diets including ovolactovegetarian (plant food sources plus milk, milk products, and eggs), lactovegetarian (plant food sources plus milk and milk products), and vegan (all plant food diet without animal foods, milk products, or eggs). Many individuals today, including professional athletes, are vegetarians for various reasons. Very active vegetarians may have difficulty getting enough protein in their diet. It is usually easier to get enough high-quality protein in your diet when consuming both animal and plant sources, but it is also possible to get all of your body's protein needs from plant sources. The following table lists some available sources.

Protein Sources for Vegetarians

Grains	Legumes	Seeds and Nuts	Vegetables
barley	dried beans	cashews	broccoli
bulgur	dried lentils	nut butters	leafy greens
cornmeal	dried peas	other nuts	
oats	peanuts	sesame seeds	
pasta	soy products	sunflower seeds	
rice		walnuts	

complete or incomplete. Incomplete proteins do not provide sufficient amounts of one or more of the essential amino acids. Complete proteins contain all of the nine essential amino acids. Foods that supply complete proteins include animal products like eggs, milk, cheese, and meat. Foods with incomplete proteins include plant food sources such as grains, nuts, vegetables, and fruits.

Vegetarians need to make sure they eat a balanced diet so that they get all of their essential amino acids. One way to do this is to mix foods like grains and legumes, because plant food sources contain varying amounts of essential amino acids, and combining certain foods that complement each other can provide the proper amino acid balance. The addition of milk products or any other animal food product results in consumption of complete proteins.

▶ Protein Requirements for Athletes

The Recommended Dietary Allowance (RDA) for the daily protein intake for active healthy adults is approximately 0.8 grams per kilogram of body weight. Certain individuals, such as growing athletes and people recovering from illness, or athletes involved in strenuous resistance training programs, can consume up to 1.6 grams per kilogram of body weight per day. There is some evidence to suggest that increasing protein intake somewhat above the RDA meets the need for improved strength and muscle mass development in athletes.

However, consuming large quantities of protein when starting a basic weight training program will not lead to rapid strength gains. The general rule is the greater the training volume and intensity, the greater the protein requirements needed to prevent a negative nitrogen balance. Generally speaking, athletes involved in high intensity, high volume training require more protein than the average person. It is important to remember that when an athlete's training program changes (reduced volume and intensity), so should the protein intake.

Consuming excessively high quantities of protein can be dangerous. A recent report by the National Research Council warns that protein intake more than two times the RDA is not recommended for anyone because of the convincing evidence that high protein intakes are associated with certain types of cancers and heart disease. Furthermore, a high protein intake places a heavy burden on the liver and kidneys to excrete excess nitrogen, and may even damage those organs.

Good sources of protein include red meat, fish, poultry, eggs, milk, cheese, nuts, dried peas, beans, bread, cereals, and vegetables. However, you should try to choose foods that are both high in protein and low in fat, such as fish, chicken, turkey, lean meats, low-fat cheese, skim milk, and egg whites (see Table 3-1).

Because the average individual living in the United States consumes more than the RDA for protein, there is no need to purchase expensive protein supplements. Nutritionists do not recommend protein supplementation for athletes, but rather eating well by following the Food Guide Pyramid.

▶ Nitrogen Balance

When an individual fails to eat an adequate amount of essential amino acids, the rate of protein synthesis (a process essential to tissue building and repair) is

TABLE 3-1
Grams of Protein Per Serving for Basic Food Exchanges

Milk—8 Grams per Serving

One Serving:	Calories:
1 cup skim milk	90
1 cup plain low-fat yogurt	90

Lean Meat—7 Grams per Serving

One Serving:	Calories:
1 ounce lean beef or pork	55
1 ounce chicken or turkey (no skin)	45
1 ounce fish, shrimp, lobster, tuna	40
1 ounce low-fat cheese	55
2 large egg whites	35

Starchy Vegetables, Breads, and Cereals—
3 Grams per Serving

One Serving:	Calories:
1/2 cup cooked or dry cereal	80
1/2 cup cooked pasta	80
1/3 cup cooked rice	80
1/2 bagel	80
1 slice bread	80
1 small baked potato	80
1/4 cup baked beans	80

Vegetables—2 Grams per Serving

One Serving:	Calories:
1/2 cup cooked vegetables	25
1 cup raw vegetables	25

Fruits— 1 Gram or Less per Serving

One Serving:	Calories:
1 small apple	60

reduced. An example of a drastic reduction in protein synthesis occurs during periods of starvation, where obvious muscle wasting and degradation is evident. During periods of reduced protein synthesis, the body is said to be in a catabolic state that results in increased excretion of nitrogen. **Nitrogen balance** is the sum of the body's nitrogen loss versus nitrogen gain. A negative nitrogen balance means that the body is in a catabolic state, indicating protein loss. A positive nitrogen balance means the body is in an anabolic state, indicating protein gain. Thus, athletes always strive to maintain an anabolic state. Eating a variety of foods and training sensibly will help maintain an anabolic state.

FAT

Fats contain more than twice as many calories (9) per gram as do carbohydrates (4). The chemical name for fat is "lipids." The main building blocks of lipids are fatty acids. Fatty acids have two classifications, saturated and unsaturated. Saturated fatty acids are heavy, more dense fats, as found in meat. Thus, saturated fatty acids are very often of animal origin. Unsaturated fatty acids are less dense and less heavy, such as liquid oil. Saturated fat sources include butter, cheese, chocolate, coconuts, oil, meats, milk, poultry; unsaturated fat sources include vegetable oil.

Fat is an important source of energy for many tissues and is the primary storage form of foods not immediately utilized by the body. This is especially important between meals. Fat deposits in the body are a fuel reserve and these deposits are stored in adipose tissue. Adipose tissue plays other roles such as supporting and protecting vital organs. However, excess amounts of adipose tissue can be harmful to your health.

According to the American Heart Association, your total daily fat intake should not exceed 30 percent of your total caloric intake. Individuals should strive to cut back on the amount of saturated fat they consume since it is associated with greater health risks. A high percentage of fat intake can result in obesity and greater risk of development of chronic diseases such as coronary heart disease. Excessive body fat may reduce athletic performance.

VITAMINS

Vitamins are non-caloric organic substances essential for building the body's cells and tissues, for proper digestion, and for energy release. Vitamins are present in small quantities in the body and function to promote many chemical reactions that occur naturally in the body. Vitamins are classified based on their solubility: fat soluble or water soluble. The fat-soluble vitamins are A, D, E, and K. The water-soluble vitamins are C and all of the B vitamins. Many vitamins serve a vital role as control agents in cell metabolism by serving as coenzymes (which assist enzymes) and as components of body tissue construction.

RDAs have been established for most vitamins. However, there is absolutely no need to take large quantities of supplemental vitamins. The preferred source of vitamins is a balanced diet. Taking large doses, also referred to as "megadoses," can be extremely harmful. All vitamins may have the potential to be toxic to the body when consumed in large quantities, but supplementation with fat-soluble vitamins usually has the most risk.

However, a standard over-the-counter multivitamin supplement with known required nutrients at RDA levels can be taken to help ensure a health-supporting diet. Also, some people may require additional vitamin supplementation, such as pregnant or lactating women, the elderly, women taking oral contraceptives, and individuals who smoke. Such decisions to take additional vitamin supplements should be discussed with a physician or registered dietition first.

MINERALS

Minerals are inorganic substances that exist freely in nature. Minerals are necessary for growth and repair of bones and teeth, metabolic activity, and function of body fluids and secretions. Minerals help in maintaining or regulating such physiological processes as muscle contraction, normal heart rhythm, and nerve impulse conduction.

As with vitamins, mineral intake may be abused. For people that are especially active and who sweat profusely for prolonged periods of time, it may be necessary to add additional salt and potassium to the diet. Both of these minerals can be easily replaced by drinking a commercially available sports drink. Ample amounts of sodium are found in many of the foods we eat, and fruits and vegetables contain high levels of potassium. Good sources of some other minerals are milk, cheese, egg yolk, and green vegetables (calcium), liver (iron), seafood and iodized salt (iodine), and milk and cheese (phosphorous).

WATER

Approximately 70 percent of the total body weight is water. Water is the most important nutrient, involved in almost every vital body process. Water is essential for maintaining the body's temperature, transporting materials, and assisting with chemical reactions. Two to three quarts of water should be ingested each day. Water levels in the body are maintained by drinking fluids, but also through the consumption of water contained in fruits, vegetables, and other foods. With excess sweating, such as during exercise and in hot, humid weather, a large amount of water is lost. In such cases, it is important to consume large quantities of water to remain hydrated.

THE FOOD GUIDE PYRAMID

The USDA **Food Guide Pyramid** (Figure 3-1) is designed to illustrate which selections of foods together give all the essential daily nutrients needed to maintain health without consuming excessive calories or fat. The Food Guide Pyramid consists of five basic food groups (levels 1–3) and the fats, oils, and sweets commonly found in our diet (level 4). The size of the food group corresponds to the recommended number of daily servings from that food group. For example, the Bread, Cereal, Rice, and Pasta Group is the largest in size (at the base of the pyramid) and it has the greatest number of recommended servings.

The circle and triangle shapes scattered throughout the pyramid's segments represent the added and naturally occurring fat and oil in certain foods (circles), as well as the added sugars (triangles). An abundance of these icons in a food group

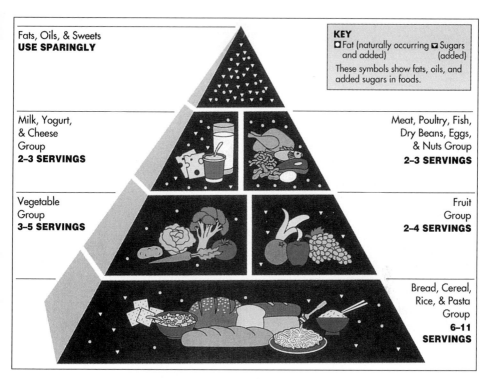

FIGURE 3-1 The USDA Food Guide Pyramid.

Level 1:   Choose plenty of foods that come from plants. Bread, cereal, rice, and pasta form the broad base of the pyramid and should make up the bulk of a health-supporting diet.

Level 2:   Also important to a health-supporting diet is an ample variety of fruits and vegetables. Fruits and vegetables provide the vitamins, minerals, carbohydrates, and fiber needed to gain and maintain strength and to stay healthy.

Level 3:   A moderate amount of lower-fat/lean foods from the Milk, Yogurt, and Cheese Group and the Meat, Poultry, Fish, Dry Beans, Eggs, and Nuts Group should be consumed on a daily basis. Dairy products provide calcium that is important for a healthy skeleton. Selections from the Meat, Poultry, Fish, Dry Beans, Eggs, and Nuts Group provide needed protein, iron, and zinc.

Level 4:   In moderation, foods containing fats, oils, and sweets can fit into a health-supporting diet. They should not, however, replace the nutrient-rich food choices found throughout Levels 1, 2, and 3.

segment indicates a large amount of naturally occurring or added fat and oil, and/or sugars. If you start at the bottom of the pyramid and work your way up, you will see how selections from the food groups can be pieced together to form a healthful overall diet.

Examples of a Serving

Bread, Cereal, Rice, and Pasta

1 slice bread
1/2 bagel or hamburger bun
1 ounce ready-to-eat cereal
1/2 cup cooked cereal, rice, or pasta

Vegetable

1 cup raw leafy vegetables
1/2 cup other vegetables, cooked or chopped raw
3/4 cup vegetable juice

Fruit

1 medium apple, banana, orange
1/2 cup chopped cooked or canned fruit
3/4 cup fruit juice

Milk, Yogurt, and Cheese

1 cup milk or yogurt
1 1/2 ounce of natural cheese
2 ounces processed cheese

Meat, Poultry, Fish, Dry Beans, Eggs, and Nuts

2–3 ounces cooked lean meat, poultry, or fish
1/2 cup cooked dry beans, 1 egg, or 2 tablespoons of peanut
butter counts as 1 ounce of lean meat

It is important to get a regular number of servings per food group for good health. The recommended number of servings per day for each food group is: 6–11 for the bread group, 3–5 for the vegetable group, 2–4 for the fruit group, 2–3 for the dairy group, and 2–3 for the meat group. The box above gives examples of what constitutes one serving.

In summary, it is important to eat a variety of lower-fat foods from among all the five groups (Levels 1, 2, and 3) each day. No one food or food group can provide all the nutrients needed for good health. Plant foods such as cereals, grains, vegetables, and fruits should comprise the basis of a health-supporting diet. Low-fat foods in the milk and meat groups should be eaten in moderation. Fats, oils, and sweets—those naturally occurring as well as those added—also need to be consumed in moderation.

NUTRITION AND ATHLETIC PERFORMANCE

GAINING WEIGHT

Gaining weight for improved athletic performance, if that is your goal, is not always an easy task. Obviously an athlete wants to gain lean body mass (muscle) and not fat mass (body fat). Any program designed to help an athlete gain weight must be accompanied by a strength training program. Each pound of increase in lean body mass requires approximately 3,500 calories of energy to support it. Adding 700 to 1,000 calories of food intake each day will support a gain of 1 to 2 pounds of lean body weight per week. Try adding an extra snack, such as a bedtime peanut butter sandwich with a glass of milk. Eat larger-than-normal portions at meal time, such as two potatoes instead of one. Eat or drink higher calorie foods, such as cran-raspberry juice instead of orange juice. Athletes may want to consult with a sports nutritionist or physician for more advice on gaining weight safely.

LOSING WEIGHT

Excess fat can limit an athlete's endurance and quickness, especially in sports such as wrestling and running. If you are concerned about your desired body weight or level of body fat, you should have your body composition measured. If weight loss is indicated, weight loss should not exceed 1 to 2 pounds per week. It is a good idea for you to keep a record of your food intake, and to become aware of what—and how much—you are eating on a daily basis. You may be quite surprised by how much you actually eat after you write it down. Try to choose foods that are lower in fat and calories. Gradual weight loss should typically be between 1 and 2 pounds per week for men and women. As previously stated, it is not recommended to lose more weight than this each week.

ACHIEVING AND MAINTAINING COMPETING WEIGHT

Athletes have used just about every technique imaginable to "make weight." A rapid decrease in weight is very unsafe immediately before or during periods of high-intensity training. Rapid weight loss can also permanently affect growth and development in young athletes. Athletes and coaches should plan training schedules based on an athlete's initial weight. Any weight loss/gain program should be carefully planned, and should be centered around a balanced diet and sensible training. Remember, frequent weight fluctuations can significantly impair athletic performance.

HIGH-CARBOHYDRATE MEALS

A healthy diet should consist of **nutrient-dense** foods. Athletes should eat lots of complex carbohydrates by following the Food Guide Pyramid. Carbohydrates are

Fitness Tip

High Protein Diets

High protein diets and protein supplements have been popular among weight trainers and bodybuilders for years. Unfortunately, most athletes need to consume no more protein than the average individual because protein intake in the U.S. is very high. Furthermore, a well-balanced diet will supply adequate amounts of protein. Protein supplementation is of no value as far as performance is concerned. Muscle growth cannot be increased by simply eating excessive amounts of high-protein foods. Athletes may need to consume higher quantities of protein during periods of high-intensity, high-volume training, but then should reduce protein intake as training schedules change. Intake of high amounts of protein beyond an athlete's caloric requirement can be stored as fat, and thus reduce athletic performance. Furthermore, high intakes of protein can lead to dehydration and loss of calcium in the body.

a very important fuel for muscular work and are needed for efficient burning of fat. As the intensity of workouts increases, so should your carbohydrate intake. Carbohydrates are stored in the muscle as glycogen. When glycogen levels are depleted, fatigue sets in. Because glycogen is the principal carbohydrate used during exercise, individuals involved in any type of training program should eat a high-carbohydrate meal one to two hours before exercise to provide fuel during exercise and after exercise to help replace the glycogen used up during exercise (see box).

SUMMARY

- Good nutritional habits will help you improve your strength and your athletic abilities.
- The six categories of nutrients are: carbohydrates, fats, protein, vitamins, minerals, and water. The first three provide energy, which is measured in calories. The latter are important for normal bodily functions.
- A good diet is composed of 50 to 60 percent carbohydrates, 25 to 30 percent fat, and 10 to 15 percent protein.
- The main function of protein is growth and repair. It is the structural basis for all body tissues. The daily protein requirement for active healthy adults is approximately 0.8 grams per kilogram of body weight. Athletes can consume up to 1.3 to 1.6 grams per kilogram of body weight per day.

Sample High-Energy, High-Carbohydrate Meal

Breakfast

1 cup orange juice or 1/2 grapefruit
1 cup hot cereal
2 eggs
3 ounces bacon, ham, or sausage
2–4 slices whole wheat toast or hot cakes with margarine
1–2 cups hot chocolate

Lunch

Clam chowder
3–6 ounces broiled fish
1/2 cup cooked rice
Green salad with dressing
2 slices bread
1–2 cups milk

Dinner

Cream of potato soup
2 pieces broiled chicken
1–2 baked potato(es)
1–2 pieces cooked broccoli
3/4 cup strawberries
1–2 cups milk

Snacks

Fruits, especially dates, raisins, apples, bananas
Milk, or a milkshake
Cookies

- There is absolutely no need to take large quantities of supplemental vitamins. In fact, this practice can be potentially dangerous. The preferred source of vitamins is a balanced diet.
- It is important that young athletes consume large quantities of water before, during, and after exercise.
- The Food Guide Pyramid makes the basics of a healthful diet easier to understand. The Food Guide Pyramid allows you to select foods that together give you all the essential nutrients you need to maintain health without eating too many calories or too much fat.

- A rapid decrease in weight is very unsafe immediately before or during periods of high-intensity training. Frequent weight fluctuations can significantly impair athletic performance.
- A pregame meal should be consumed one to two hours before competition.
- Muscle growth cannot be increased by eating high-protein foods. Intake of high amounts of protein beyond an athlete's caloric requirement will only be stored as fat. Furthermore, high intakes of protein can lead to dehydration and loss of calcium in the body.

▶ **Carbohydrates   p. 25**
Organic compounds composed of one or more sugars that are derived from plant sources.

▶ **Essential Amino Acids   p. 26**
A group of nine amino acids that cannot be made by the body and thus must be obtained from food.

▶ **Fats   p. 29**
Organic compounds that are composed of glycerol and fatty acids.

▶ **Food Guide Pyramid   p. 30**
A diagram that shows the proper selections of foods together with all the essential daily nutrients needed to maintain health without consuming excessive calories or fat.

▶ **Minerals   p. 30**
Inorganic substances that are necessary for growth and repair of bones and teeth, metabolic activity, and function of body fluids and secretions.

▶ **Nitrogen Balance   p. 28**
The sum of the body's nitrogen loss versus nitrogen gain.

▶ **Nonessential Amino Acids   p. 26**
A group of eleven amino acids that the body can make.

▶ **Nutrient Density   p. 33**
A measure that compares a food's nutrient value to its energy value. When the contribution to nutrient needs exceeds that to energy needs, the food is a nutrient-dense source of that nutrient.

▶ **Protein   p. 26**
A food substance formed from amino acids.

▶ **Vitamins   p. 29**
Organic compounds found in food that are essential to normal metabolism.

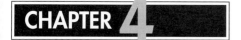

CHAPTER 4

TRAINING PRINCIPLES FOR A SUCCESSFUL PROGRAM

OBJECTIVES

After reading this chapter, you should be able to do the following:

- Define basic weight training principles.
- Utilize common weight training terms.
- Recognize signs of overtraining.
- Understand and list safety considerations in the weight room.

KEY TERMS

While reading this chapter, you will become familiar with the following terms:

- ► Frequency
- ► Load
- ► One-Repetition Maximum (1RM)
- ► Overload Principle
- ► Powerlifting
- ► Principle of Reversibility
- ► Principle of Specificity
- ► Progression
- ► Repetition
- ► Rest
- ► Set
- ► Volume

BASIC TRAINING PRINCIPLES

There are probably hundreds of different weight training systems. Most of these systems are based on the **overload principle.** The overload principle states that a muscle or system will adapt (increase in strength or aerobic power) when it is stressed to overcome greater stresses than it is normally used to. When the stresses are too great, the body reacts negatively (i.e., reduced immune function, injury and fatigue). When training ceases, improvements in physiological parameters are quickly lost. Running 3 miles or lifting 75 pounds per day will produce an overload response for only so long, then further gains will be minimal.

The overload principle is based in part on the research of Dr. Hans Selye. Selye identified a pattern of physical stress referred to as the general adaptation syndrome (GAS). The GAS reveals how the human body responds and adapts to physical stress over time. Initially, a stress to the body causes the body to respond and adapt to that stress. With exercise, muscles get stronger and the heart and lungs work more efficiently, which are both signs of adaptation to training. When the stress is too great for too long, the body is not able to respond adequately, and the stress leads to exhaustion. Athletes should be well aware of the common signs and symptoms of overtraining.

When muscles are overloaded, they adapt by getting stronger and larger. When the exercise stimulus is removed, the training adaptations reverse—meaning, "use it or lose it." This phenomenon is referred to as the **principle of reversibility.** If you do not remain on a maintenance program, improvements in strength and/or aerobic endurance will gradually diminish.

Muscle mass also declines with age, resulting in decreased muscular strength and endurance. For each decade after the age of twenty-five, 3 to 5 percent of muscle mass is lost. Such losses with age are primarily due to lack of regular physical activity. A regular exercise program can reduce many of the effects of normal aging.

Another important training principle is the **principle of specificity.** If you want to be a world-class swimmer, what do you do? You swim! Training programs should be designed with specific goals and objectives in mind. For the majority of people starting a strength training program, specificity does not seem that important. However, as training progresses, specificity becomes more important. If you want to develop explosive power, you will want to lift a great deal of weight using few repetitions. On the other hand, if muscular endurance is more important, a program involving light weights with higher repetitions should be stressed. It is important to work all the major muscle groups on a regular basis.

COMMON WEIGHT TRAINING TERMS

The **load** is the amount of resistance or weight used. When using free weights, the weight is the load. When performing calisthenics, such as pull-ups, your body weight serves as the load. Before the load is increased, a solid base of training should be established. Proper technique should always be demonstrated before any load is utilized. Once proper technique has been demonstrated, load can gradually be applied until eight to ten repetitions can be performed in a set.

The quantity of exercise performed in a given time period is the **volume.** The greater the training volume, the greater the demands on the body. Training volume is influenced by frequency, load, sets, and repetitions. When first starting out, it is a good idea to keep training volume low, and gradually increase it over time. Performing overly high-volume workouts (i.e. too much weight lifted repeatedly and frequently) can lead to overtraining and injury.

Repetitions refers to the number of times an exercise is performed per each exercise session or set. In resistance training, you should initially perform eight to ten repetitions for upper body exercises and ten to twelve for lower body exercises. However, there is no absolute number of repetitions that should be performed. Once the predetermined maximum number of repetitions per set is achieved, both the weight and the maximum number of repetitions can be increased.

A **set** is the number of times a particular exercise is performed during the workout. Generally one to three sets of eight to ten different resistance training exercises should be performed. Some weight training equipment is designed so that you perform only one set per exercise. However, most training programs involve at least two sets per exercise. The first set is often performed at a lighter weight, while the second and third sets may use heavier weights. The first set serves as a warm-up. In the early stages of training, one to two sets of each exercise should be performed.

Rest is the amount of time between sets or training sessions. Individuals should be encouraged to rest for the same amount of time it took to perform the exercise. Thus, if an exercise takes thirty seconds to perform, rest thirty seconds before starting the next exercise. Rest periods vary between running intervals, from several seconds to several minutes depending on the distance run and workout goals. Shorter rest periods place a greater demand on the body to adapt, so longer rest periods may be necessary for the beginner. It is always a good idea to take a day off between weight training sessions, especially in the beginning.

Fitness Tip

Making Good Use of Time During Workouts

When time is limited—let's say for example that you need to complete an entire workout in thirty minutes—try working another body part while resting the body area just worked. For example, immediately following an upper body exercise, perform a lower body exercise before repeating another upper body exercise. This way, you will be able to rest exercised body areas between sets while maximizing your time in the gym.

Frequency refers to the number of training sessions per week. A frequency of two to three exercise sessions per week is recommended, followed by at least one day of rest between workouts, for most health-related training. Of course, some athletes train six to seven days a week, sometimes two or three times per day. Such frequency of training could lead to overtraining, especially in the inexperienced lifter.

Progression refers to how quickly changes are made in a workout. A gradual addition of weight or intensity within your capabilities allows the body to adapt physically to a higher workload. Many people starting out with a resistance or endurance training program will try to lift or exercise too much early on in their training program. Such practices often lead to injuries and chronic fatigue. To maintain maximal stimulus, the resistance and/or number of repetitions must be increased periodically. Once an individual is able to lift the preestablished number of repetitions, a small (5 to 10%) increase in resistance can be made. When the weight being lifted is increased, the number of repetitions should be reduced (i.e., if the preestablished number of repetitions was twelve, after an increase in weight a new repetition maximum might be seven or eight). As the individual adjusts to the new training stimulus, he will soon be able to lift the new weight twelve times, at which point a new weight and repetition maximum should be established.

ADVANCED STRENGTH TRAINING TECHNIQUES

Powerlifting generally involves core weight lifting exercises, such as the bench press, squat, and deadlift. These types of exercises are commonly used by athletes to develop overall strength and explosive power. Powerlifting is effective, but can also be dangerous if not performed correctly. Individuals should be gradually introduced to powerlifting.

The **one-repetition maximum (1RM)** is used to establish starting weights for different exercises. It involves an individual lifting the maximum amount of weight he or she can lift for a particular exercise. Once an individual's 1RM is established, different percentages of the 1RM weight are used when performing selected exercises. (Determining your 1RM is discussed in more detail in chapter 5.)

Weight Training Progression Guidelines

- Increase the resistance, repetitions, sets, or rest periods one at a time.
- Increase the number of repetitions before increasing the resistance.
- When making an increase in resistance, decrease the number of repetitions.
- To increase muscular endurance, decrease the rest intervals between sets.
- Make conservative adjustments in progression over time.

OVERTRAINING

Overtraining occurs when performance in athletics or training remains constant or decreases over time. Usually overtraining is caused by poor program design, lack of adequate rest, and failure to keep a training log. Training sessions should be planned carefully so that the workout intensity increases gradually and the individual has adequate time to rest. The following conditions can be signs of overtraining:

- Loss of body weight
- Decreased appetite
- Muscle soreness that does not go away, even after rest
- Increased illness, such as colds, flu, etc.
- Constipation or diarrhea
- Decreased performance
- Lack of desire in training or competing

SAFETY CONSIDERATIONS

Safety is always the first concern for anyone working out with weights. Lifting weights can cause serious injury if basic safety rules are not followed. By simply using good common sense, and following the rules outlined on p. 42, your workout will be safer and more effective.

KEEPING TRACK OF YOUR PROGRESS

It is important to keep track of your progress. After each workout, record the number of sets and repetitions performed. Also make notes about how you felt, if you were tired or rested, if a particular exercise caused you more problems than others, or if you had a new pain. A training log will help you train "smart." This log need not be exotic and can consist of simply writing down exercises, sets, reps, weight, and how you felt on any given day. You may buy a custom made log or simply make your own with an inexpensive store bought notebook.

SUMMARY

- Almost all weight training systems are based on the overload principle, which states that a muscle or system will adapt (increase in strength or aerobic power) when it is stressed to overcome greater stresses than it is normally used to.
- Training programs should always be designed with specific goals in mind.
- When individuals do not remain active or stop training, gains in strength and/or aerobic endurance are lost.

Fitness Tip

Safety in the Weight Room

- Always be aware of everything that is going on around you in the weight room.
- When beginning a weight training program, avoid single or maximal lifts, sudden explosive movements, or competing against others.
- Do not try to show off. Never lift more weight than you are capable of.
- Always use collars with free weights.
- Work out with a partner when lifting free weights and take turns spotting.
- When lifting a weight up off the floor, keep it close to your body. Lift with your legs, not your back.
- Progress gradually and within your limits. Overtraining predisposes you to injuries.
- Exhale during the lifting part of the movement and inhale during the recovery phase.
- Do not use any equipment that is broken or damaged, or which you do not fit in properly.
- Rest between sets of each exercise and between exercises.
- All strength training workouts should be preceded by a warm-up period and followed by a cool-down period.
- If any soreness, fatigue, or pain is noticed before a workout, the workout should be modified or canceled if necessary.

- Before the load (volume and intensity or actual weight lifted) is increased, a solid base of training should be established.
- The greater the training volume (sets × reps), the greater the demands on the body.
- Initially, individuals should perform eight to ten repetitions for upper body exercises and ten to twelve for lower body exercises.
- Generally one to three sets of eight to ten different resistance training exercises should be performed.
- Individuals should be encouraged to rest body areas between resistance training exercises.
- A frequency of two to three strength training sessions per week is recommended, followed by at least one day of rest between workouts, for most health-related training.
- Too much exercise in the early stages of a training program can lead to injuries and chronic fatigue.

- Powerlifting is effective, but can also be dangerous if not performed correctly.
- Overtraining occurs when performance in athletics or training remains constant or decreases over time. Usually overtraining is caused by poor program design, lack of adequate rest, and failure to keep a training log.
- Safety is always the first concern for anyone working out with weights. Lifting weights can cause serious injury if basic safety rules are not followed.
- It is important to keep track of your progress. After each workout, record the number of sets and repetitions you performed.

► **Frequency   p. 40**
The number of training sessions per week.

► **Load   p. 38**
The amount of resistance or weight used.

► **One-Repetition Maximum (1RM)   p. 40**
A procedure used to establish starting weights for different exercises. It involves an individual lifting the maximum amount of weight he or she can lift for a particular exercise.

► **Overload Principle   p. 38**
A muscle or system will adapt when it is stressed to overcome greater stresses than it is normally used to.

► **Powerlifting   p. 40**
A type of weight lifting designed to develop overall strength and explosive power that generally involves core weight lifting exercises such as the bench press, squat, and deadlift.

► **Principle of Reversibility   p. 38**
When the exercise stimulus is removed, the training adaptations reverse.

► **Principle of Specificity   p. 38**
The exercise(s) chosen for a training program should reflect the desired outcome.

► **Progression   p. 40**
How quickly changes are made in a workout.

► **Repetitions   p. 39**
The number of times an exercise is performed per exercise session or set.

► **Rest   p. 39**
The amount of time between sets and training sessions.

► **Set   p. 39**
The number of times a particular exercise is performed during the workout.

► **Volume   p. 39**
The quantity of exercise performed in a given time period.

CHAPTER 5

DESIGNING A PROGRAM THAT'S RIGHT FOR YOU

OBJECTIVES

After reading this chapter, you should be able to do the following:

- Describe a variety of weight training programs.
- Know how to choose a weight training gym.
- Understand how to determine your baseline strength levels.

KEY TERMS

While reading this chapter, you will become familiar with the following terms:

▶ Forced Repetitions to Failure

▶ Periodization

▶ Pyramid System

▶ Split Routine System

▶ Super Set System

PROGRAM DESIGN CONSIDERATIONS

There are a variety of ways to design a weight training program. Virtually all strength and weight training systems are based on a variation of the fundamental principles of strength and weight training: load, repetition, intensity, rest, and frequency.

Before you start a strength and weight training program, you need to determine what your individual goals are. Do you want to get bigger, lose weight, or run faster? Your training program should reflect your desired goals. Remember, specific training programs can be designed to meet your individual goals no matter what they might be. A proper initial program will help you attain the desired results.

FREE WEIGHTS VS. MACHINES

There are pros and cons to both free weights and machines. The major pros regarding free weights are the cost, convenience, and exercise variety. In addition, free weights are generally the preferred choice of equipment among athletes because they improve balance and coordination as well as strength. One of the major concerns with free weights is safety. Free weights hold many more opportunities for injury than do machines. To minimize risk when lifting free weights, always follow the guidelines listed in the Fitness Tip.

The major pros of machines are their safety and ease of use, and the speed in which a complete upper and lower body workout can be achieved. Many people today simply do not have time to lift weights four or five times a week for an hour each time. Most weight lifting machines are designed in a manner that allows the individual to get an upper and lower body workout in thirty to forty-five minutes.

Fitness Tip

Free Weight Safety Guidelines

- Always use collars.
- Always work out with a partner.
- Put weight plates away when finished.
- Do not show off; never lift more weight than you are capable of.
- When lifting a weight up off the floor, make sure to keep it close to your body.
- Use a weight belt for lifts that place stress on the lower back (i.e., squats).

FINDING THE RIGHT FACILITY

One of the most important factors to consider when choosing a health club is what you expect to get out of the club. If your goal is to become a nationally ranked bodybuilder, you should look for specific clubs in your area that specialize in servicing such clients. If your goal is to get a quick total body workout in the shortest amount of time, you should consider clubs that specialize in that service. Before going shopping, know what you are shopping for. The Fitness Tip will help you prepare to find a gym that is right for you.

Fitness Tip

Some Things to Consider When Choosing a Gym

- Join a gym near your home. The closer the gym, the more likely you will get there.
- Choose a club with a friendly atmosphere. Don't join a "singles" club or a bodybuilders club if you don't like that type of atmosphere.
- Carefully check the cost of membership. Most of the negative press around health clubs in the last ten years has come from deceptive advertising.
- Know what type of membership options are available. For example, if you work from 3:00 P.M. to 11:00 P.M. and prefer to work out late at night, check into the availability of an off-hours-rate membership.
- Get a free trial workout. Even the best deal is not worth it if you don't like the facility or staff.
- Check out the equipment. Is the equipment well maintained and new? If you just want to lift free weights and don't care about machines, there may be smaller, less costly gyms available.
- Visit the club at different hours. See what the crowds are like at different times of the day.
- Examine the contract carefully. Make sure you know what you're getting for your money and how long and how much your monetary commitment will be. What are the penalties for breaking a contract? What is the method of payment?
- Ask about the club's employees. Are they trained and certified?
- Go with your "gut" instinct. If you think something is fishy, it probably is.

Adapted from *Consumer Reports* (January 1996).

ESTABLISHING YOUR BASELINE STRENGTH

Another thing to consider before you get started with your weight training program is the need to assess your baseline strength. Training programs are designed to progressively add weight to each exercise you perform so that you continue to develop and maintain strength. Without knowing your baseline strength level you risk lifting more than you should, which can lead to injury, or not enough, which can delay your improvements. There are two different types of strength assessment: isotonic and muscular endurance.

Isotonic, or dynamic, strength is typically measured by the maximum amount of weight that can be lifted one time [one-repetition maximum (1RM)] or the number of repetitions that can be performed at a selected percentage of 1RM (10RM). This corresponds to a weight that can be lifted a maximum of ten times. Muscular endurance is measured with a variety of calisthenics and generally requires no equipment.

▶ Baseline Measure of Isotonic Strength

Athletes determine their baseline strength via a test called the one-repetition maximum, or 1RM. With this test, the athlete performs a variety of lifts with different amounts of weight until they find a weight they can lift only once. Once this weight has been established for a particular exercise, different percentages of the weight are used to develop the workout. For example, if an athlete's 1RM for the bench press is 100 lbs., she might start out performing the exercise at 60 percent intensity level (60 lbs.) for three sets.

An easier and safer way to determine the correct starting weight is to estimate your 1RM. With this technique, individuals start out by performing an exercise ten times with a particular weight. This process is repeated, either adding or reducing weight, until a weight that can only be lifted ten times is found. This method of establishing the starting weight is referred to as the 10-repetition maximum, or 10RM. Assessment 5-1 at the end of this chapter will help you estimate your 1RM. Once the 1RM is estimated, a training program can be developed using different percentages of the 1RM. The initial starting weight should be changed if chronic fatigue is noticed one to two days later. The 10RM test must be repeated on a regular basis to reestablish new 1RMs as training adaptations occur.

▶ Baseline Measure of Muscular Endurance

As discussed in earlier chapters, muscular endurance is the ability of a muscle or muscle group to perform repeated contractions for an extended period of time, whereas muscular strength is defined as the greatest amount of force a muscle or group of muscles can produce during one maximal contraction. Muscular endurance can be assessed with a variety of calisthenics. Muscular strength and endurance are specific to the muscle group being tested, and thus there is no single test available to assess total body muscular strength or endurance. It is recommended that a variety of muscular strength and endurance tests be performed so that a fair assessment of upper and lower body fitness is determined. Assessments 5-2 and 5-3 include additional tests to measure muscular endurance.

GENERAL TRAINING SYSTEMS

As discussed in chapter 4, most strength and weight training systems are based on the overload principle. You may recall that the overload principle states that a muscle will adapt (increase in strength) when it is stressed to overcome more stress than it is used to. To illustrate the overload principle, imagine that you can bench press 100 lbs. for three sets of ten repetitions. For the next six months you lift that same weight for the same number of repetitions three days a week. At the end of six months, will you be much stronger than you were two weeks to a month after starting your program? Probably not. This is because your muscles adapted to the initial weight and would have to be challenged with greater weight (overload) if greater strength gains were desired.

When starting out it is important to begin with a basic program and modify it with time and training experience. Which system you use will depend on your specific goals, experience, and the type of equipment available to you. Once you get a base of training established and are comfortable with your training, vary your routine occasionally. The following box offers an example of a basic weight training program.

A sensible strength training program for general conditioning should consist of two to three days of strength training and thirty to forty minutes of cardiovascular conditioning (running, swimming, cycling, etc.) three days per week. If you are involved in athletics you will want to reduce the intensity and frequency of your strength training program during the competitive season. It is a good idea to get guidelines from your coach regarding your strength training program before, during, and after an athletic season. Otherwise, if you are involved in a strength and conditioning program for overall conditioning and health, try to stay with your program all year long.

PERIODIZATION SYSTEM

Periodization is a technique used by virtually all athletes. Periodization is a way to systematically plan your training sessions to avoid overtraining and to maximize your workout sessions. With periodization, athletes vary the type, amount, and intensity of training for several weeks, a month, or a whole year. Periodization phases can be broken into off-season, preseason and in-season training. During the off-season training period the volume and intensity of weight training is high. During the preseason phase volume may decrease but the intensity stays the same or increases. During the competitive season both the volume and intensity of weight training generally are reduced.

A Basic Weight Training Program

How long: 45–60 minutes
How often: 3 days per week
How many: 2 to 3 sets of each exercise as per program goals and weight chosen

Exercises

To develop the chest

1. Bench press (barbell)
2. Dumbbell fly
3. Push-up

To develop the shoulders

1. Dumbbell shoulder press
2. Dumbbell lateral raise
3. Pull-up

To develop the arms

1. Triceps extension
2. One-arm French curl
3. Seated or standing dumbbell curl

To develop the upper and lower back

1. Upright rowing (barbell)
2. Upright rowing (dumbbells)
3. Shoulder shrug
4. Lat pull (machine)
5. Pull-up
6. Abdominals (crunches)
7. Back extension

To develop the lower body

1. Lunge
2. Calf raise
3. Knee extension (machine)
4. Hamstring curl (machine)

Periodization allows you to perform the same or similar exercises each training session while still varying the workout. This technique allows your body to adapt rapidly, without increased risk of injury. Start by making a schedule of your workouts for one month. An example of a periodization schedule for one month follows.

Week one:	**Low intensity, high volume**
	Upper body exercise: 4 sets of 10 reps
	Exercise example: bench press (80 lbs.)
	Lower body exercise: 4 sets of 15 reps
	Exercise example: knee extension (50 lbs.)
Week two:	**Medium intensity, high volume**
	Bench press: 4 sets of 10 reps (90 lbs.)
	Knee extension: 4 sets of 15 reps (60 lbs.)
Week three:	**High intensity, low volume**
	Bench press: 3 sets of 8 reps (100 lbs.)
	Knee extension: 3 sets of 10 reps (70 lbs.)
Week four:	**Low intensity, high volume**
	Bench press: 4 sets of 10 reps (80 lbs.)
	Knee extension: 4 sets of 15 reps (50 lbs.)

PYRAMID SYSTEM

The **pyramid system** has become a popular technique among athletes and body-builders. With this system an individual performs continuous sets of exercises, progressing from light to heavy resistance while decreasing the number of repetitions. For example, an athlete who can lift a 25 lb. dumbbell ten times comfortably might structure his sets for this exercise as follows:

First set: 10 reps, 25 lbs.
Second set: 8 reps, 30 lbs.
Third set: 6 reps, 35 lbs.
Fourth set: 8 to 10 reps, 20 lbs.

In the first three sets of this pyramid system the weight is increased while the number of repetitions is decreased. The final set uses a lighter weight and increased repetitions for the cool-down.

SPLIT ROUTINE SYSTEM

A **split routine system** trains different body parts on alternate days in an effort to stimulate hypertrophy of all muscles in a particular area of the body. A typical training routine might work the chest, shoulders, and back on Monday, Wednesday, and Friday, and the arms, legs, and abdominal muscles on Tuesday, Thursday, and Saturday. Split routines can vary as well. Instead of a six-day training routine, you can develop a four-day training routine. Split routines allow you to work a particular part of the body one day and rest that area the next day while you work another body area. Split routine training is not recommended for children because the volume and intensity of training may be too strenuous.

SUPER SET SYSTEM

With the **super set system,** opposing muscle groups are worked through exercises performed one right after another. An example of a super set workout would be to perform biceps curls immediately followed by triceps extensions, or leg extensions immediately followed by leg curls. Super setting is a popular way to increase muscle hypertrophy.

FORCED REPETITIONS TO FAILURE

Forced repetitions to failure is a technique performed with a training partner. The training partner helps the lifter only enough to complete the movement. This technique is not recommended for beginners. Such high-intensity training routines should only be incorporated after a solid base of training has been established.

TRAINING FOR SPORT AND PERFORMANCE

A training routine for sport and performance differs from a general conditioning program in that it is more specific. Each sport has its own unique physical demands. The soccer player needs a great deal of body strength and endurance, while the tennis player needs a great deal of arm strength and endurance as well as leg endurance. It is important to focus on the specific muscle groups utilized in a particular sport and develop your training program around exercises that will strengthen those muscle groups. Chapter 13 outlines detailed training programs using a variety of training techniques for a selection of sports.

▶ **Forced Repetitions to Failure   p. 51**
A technique in which a training partner helps the lifter only enough to complete a particular exercise movement.

▶ **Periodization   p. 48**
A way to systematically plan your training sessions to avoid overtraining and to maximize your workout sessions by varying the type, amount, and intensity of training for several weeks, a month, or a whole year.

▶ **Pyramid System   p. 50**
Performing continuous sets of exercises, progressing from light to heavy resistance, while decreasing the number of repetitions along the way.

▶ **Split Routine System   p. 50**
Training different body parts on alternate days in an effort to stimulate hypertrophy of all muscles in a particular area of the body.

▶ **Super Set System   p. 51**
Training opposing muscle groups through exercises performed one right after another.

SUMMARY

- Virtually all strength and weight training systems are based on a variation of the fundamental principles of strength and weight training (load, repetition, intensity, rest, and frequency).
- Training with free weights is inexpensive and convenient, and it provides a great deal of variety.
- The major benefits of training with machines are safety, ease of use, and shortened workout time.
- Perhaps the most important factor to consider when looking for a health club is what you expect to get out of the club.
- Before you start your weight training program you should assess your initial level of strength using the 1RM method or the 10RM method.
- Most strength and weight training systems are based on the basic principle of overload.
- It is important to begin with a basic program and modify it with time and training experience.
- A sensible strength training program for general conditioning should consist of two to three days of strength training and at least thirty to forty minutes of cardiovascular conditioning (running, swimming, cycling, etc.) three days per week.
- Periodization is a way to systematically plan your training sessions to avoid overtraining and to maximize your workout sessions by varying the type, amount, and intensity of training for several weeks, a month, or a whole year.
- The pyramid system is a technique in which individuals perform continuous sets of exercises progressing from light to heavy resistance while decreasing the number of repetitions.
- A split routine system trains different body parts on alternate days in an effort to stimulate hypertrophy of all muscles in a particular area of the body.
- The super set system is a technique that trains opposing muscle groups through exercises performed one right after another.
- Forced repetitions to failure is a technique in which a training partner helps the lifter only enough to complete a particular exercise movement. This technique is not recommended for beginners.

Assessment 5-1

Name   Section   Date

Suggested Exercises for 1RM Testing

Machine	Free Weights
Leg press	Squat
Bench press	Bench press
Lat pulldown	Deadlift
Shoulder press	Military press
Triceps pressdown	Close grip bench
Arm curl	EZ curl

Procedure:

1. You should be rested and adequately warmed-up.
2. A partner should be available to assist.
3. Start off with a weight that is comfortable and perform one repetition.
4. Either add weight or take weight off depending on how hard or easy the exercise was.
5. Wait at least two to four minutes before making another attempt.
6. Continue the process until a weight allowing only ten repetitions is discovered.
7. See Table 5-1 to find the weight you achieved and then find the weight on the same line in the 1RM column to estimate your 1RM.

Note: Be certain that proper spotting techniques are used (i.e., two to three spotters on maximum bench and squat, one spotter on each end and one behind the lifter). An adequate warm-up consisting of a general, overall body warm-up lasting five to ten minutes and two to three light and medium sets on each exercise, that will be tested, should precede any maximal testing.

TABLE 5-1
Estimating One-Repetition Maximum (1RM)

Wt. Lbs.	50%	52.5%	55%	57.5%	60%	62.5%	65%	67.5%	70%	72%	75%	77%	80%	82%	85%	87%	90%	92%	95%	97%
200	100	105	110	115	120	125	130	135	140	145	150	155	160	165	170	175	180	185	190	195
210	105	110	115	120	125	130	135	140	145	150	160	165	170	175	180	185	190	195	200	205
220	110	115	120	125	130	140	145	150	155	160	165	170	175	180	185	195	200	205	210	215
230	115	120	125	130	140	145	150	155	160	165	170	180	185	190	195	200	205	210	220	225
240	120	125	130	140	145	150	160	165	170	175	180	185	190	200	205	210	215	220	230	235
250	125	130	135	145	150	155	160	170	175	180	190	195	200	205	210	220	225	230	240	245
260	130	135	140	150	155	160	170	175	180	190	195	200	210	215	220	230	235	240	245	255
270	135	140	145	155	160	170	175	180	190	195	200	210	215	225	230	235	245	250	255	265
280	140	145	150	160	170	175	180	190	195	205	210	215	225	230	240	245	250	260	265	275
290	145	150	160	165	175	180	190	195	205	210	220	225	230	240	245	255	260	270	275	285
300	150	160	165	170	180	190	195	200	210	220	225	235	240	250	255	265	270	280	285	295
310	155	165	170	180	185	195	200	210	215	225	230	240	250	255	265	270	280	285	295	300
320	160	170	175	185	190	200	210	215	225	230	240	250	255	265	270	280	290	295	305	310
330	165	175	180	190	200	205	215	220	230	240	250	255	265	270	280	290	295	305	315	320
340	170	180	185	195	205	215	220	230	240	245	255	265	270	280	290	300	305	315	325	330
350	175	185	190	200	210	220	230	235	245	255	260	270	280	290	300	305	315	325	330	340
360	180	190	200	205	215	225	235	245	250	260	270	280	290	295	305	315	325	335	340	350
370	185	195	205	215	220	230	240	250	260	270	280	285	295	305	315	325	330	340	350	360
380	190	200	210	220	230	240	245	255	265	275	285	295	305	315	325	335	340	350	360	370
390	195	205	215	225	235	245	255	265	275	285	295	300	310	320	330	340	350	360	370	380

% of 1RM Repetitions

Weight Lifted (lb.)

% of 1RM Repetitions

Wt. Lbs.	50%	52.5%	55%	57.5%	60%	62.5%	65%	67.5%	70%	72%	75%	77%	80%	82%	85%	87%	90%	92%	95%	97%
400	200	210	220	230	240	250	260	270	280	290	300	310	320	330	340	350	360	370	380	390
410	205	215	225	235	245	255	265	275	285	295	310	320	330	340	350	360	370	380	390	400
420	210	220	230	240	250	265	275	285	295	305	315	325	335	345	360	370	380	390	400	410
430	215	225	235	245	260	270	280	290	300	310	320	335	345	355	365	375	390	400	410	420
440	220	230	240	255	265	275	285	295	310	320	330	340	350	365	375	385	395	405	420	430
450	225	235	250	260	270	280	290	305	315	325	340	350	360	370	380	395	405	415	430	440
460	230	240	255	265	275	290	300	310	320	335	345	355	370	380	390	405	415	425	440	450
470	235	245	260	270	280	295	305	315	330	340	350	365	375	390	400	410	425	435	445	460
480	240	250	265	275	290	300	310	325	335	350	360	370	385	395	410	420	430	445	455	470
490	245	255	270	280	295	305	320	330	345	355	370	380	390	405	415	430	440	455	465	480
500	250	265	275	290	300	315	325	340	350	365	375	390	400	415	425	440	450	465	475	490
510	255	270	280	295	305	320	330	345	360	370	385	395	410	420	435	445	460	470	485	495
520	260	275	285	300	310	325	340	350	365	375	390	405	415	430	440	455	470	480	495	505
530	265	280	290	305	320	330	345	360	370	385	400	410	425	435	450	465	475	490	505	515
540	270	285	295	310	325	340	350	365	380	390	405	420	430	445	460	475	485	500	515	525
550	275	290	300	315	330	345	360	370	385	400	410	425	440	455	470	480	495	510	520	535
560	280	295	310	320	335	350	365	380	390	405	420	435	450	460	475	490	500	515	530	545
570	285	300	315	330	340	355	370	385	400	415	430	440	455	470	485	500	515	525	540	555
580	290	305	320	335	350	365	375	390	405	420	435	450	465	480	490	505	520	535	550	565
590	295	310	325	340	355	370	385	400	415	430	440	455	470	485	500	515	530	545	560	575

Weight Lifted (lb.)

TABLE 5-1
(continued)

Wt. Lbs.	50%	52.5%	55%	57.5%	60%	62.5%	65%	67.5%	70%	72%	75%	77%	80%	82%	85%	87%	90%	92%	95%	97%
600	300	315	330	345	360	375	390	405	420	435	450	465	480	495	510	525	540	555	570	585
610	305	320	335	350	365	380	395	410	425	440	460	475	490	505	520	535	550	565	580	595
620	310	325	340	355	370	390	405	420	435	450	465	480	495	510	530	545	560	575	590	605
630	315	330	345	360	380	395	410	425	440	455	470	490	505	520	535	550	570	585	600	615
640	320	335	350	370	385	400	415	430	450	465	480	495	510	530	545	560	575	590	610	625
650	325	340	355	375	390	405	420	440	455	470	485	505	520	535	550	570	585	600	615	635
660	330	345	360	380	395	415	430	445	460	480	495	510	530	545	560	580	595	610	625	645
670	335	350	370	385	400	420	435	450	470	485	500	520	535	555	570	585	605	620	635	655
680	340	355	375	390	410	425	440	460	475	495	510	525	545	560	580	595	610	630	645	665
690	345	360	380	395	415	430	450	465	485	500	515	535	550	570	585	605	620	640	655	675
700	350	370	385	405	420	440	455	475	490	510	525	545	560	580	595	615	630	650	665	685
710	355	375	390	410	425	445	460	480	495	515	530	550	570	585	605	620	640	655	675	690
720	360	380	395	415	430	450	470	485	505	520	540	560	575	595	610	630	650	665	685	700
730	365	385	400	420	440	455	475	495	510	530	550	565	585	600	620	640	655	675	695	710
740	370	390	405	425	445	465	480	500	520	535	555	575	590	610	630	650	665	685	700	720
750	375	395	415	430	450	470	490	505	525	545	560	580	600	620	640	655	675	695	710	730

% of 1RM Repetitions

Weight Lifted (lb.)

Assessment 5-2

Push-Up Test

Name _____ Section _____ Date _____

This activity is best performed with a partner if possible.

1. Lie on your stomach on a padded floor. Your body should be straight and your hands should be shoulder width apart (Figure 5-1). Use the modified push-up position if you have very poor upper body strength or low back problems. For the modified push-up test, pull your feet up off the ground while keeping your knees on the floor (Figure 5-2).
2. After a warm-up period, raise up until your arms are straight and then return to the starting position. It is important to keep your upper body rigid throughout the complete movement. Your chest should come within 3 inches of the floor.
3. Count the total number of push-ups performed until exhaustion.
4. Compare your score to the norms listed in Table 5-2.
5. Perform this test every two to three months and track your progress.

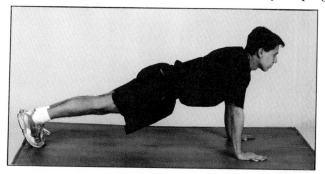

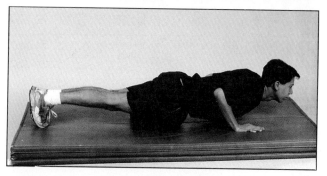

FIGURE 5-1 Push-ups.

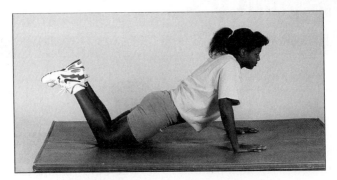

FIGURE 5-2 Modified push-ups.

TABLE 5-2
Norms for the Push-Up Test

Age Group:	20–29	30–39	40–49	50–59	60+
Men					
Excellent	>55	>45	>40	>35	>30
Good	45–54	35–44	30–39	25–34	20–29
Average	35–44	25–34	20–29	15–24	10–19
Fair	20–34	15–24	12–19	8–14	5–9
Poor	<19	<14	<11	<7	<4
Women					
Excellent	>49	>40	>35	>30	>20
Good	34–48	25–39	20–34	15–29	5–19
Average	17–33	12–24	8–19	6–14	3–4
Fair	6–16	4–11	3–7	2–5	1–2
Poor	<5	<3	<2	<1	<0

From Pollock & Wilmore (1990). Exercise in Health and Disease, W. B. Saunders Co., Philadelphia, 1990.

	Test 1	Test 2	Test 3	Test 4	Test 5	Test 6
Date						
Number of Push-Ups						
Rating (From Table 5-2)						

Assessment 5-3

Bent-Knee Sit-Up Test

Name   Section   Date

This activity is best performed with a partner.

1. Lie on your back on a padded floor. Bend your knees and place your feet flat on the floor 12 to 18 inches from the buttocks.
2. Interlock your hands behind your neck.
3. Have your partner hold your feet down.
4. When your partner says "go," try to perform as many sit-ups as possible in sixty seconds. Rising from a lying position up to the point where the elbows touch the knees and returning to the starting position equals one complete sit-up (Figure 5-3).
5. Record the number of complete sit-ups. Consult Table 5-3 to determine your performance.

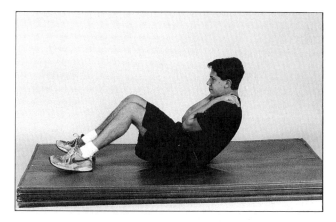

FIGURE 5-3 Bent-knee sit-ups.

TABLE 5-3
Norms for the Timed Bent-Knee Sit-Up Test

Age Group:	20–29	30–39	40–49	50–59	60+
Men					
Excellent	>48	>40	>35	>30	>25
Good	43–47	35–39	30–34	25–29	20–24
Average	37–42	29–34	24–29	19–24	14–19
Fair	33–36	25–28	20–23	15–18	10–13
Poor	<32	<24	<19	<14	<9
Women					
Excellent	>44	>36	>31	>26	>21
Good	39–43	31–35	26–30	21–25	16–20
Average	33–38	25–30	19–25	15–20	10–15
Fair	29–32	21–24	16–18	11–14	6–9
Poor	<28	<20	<15	<10	<5

From Pollock & Wilmore (1990). *Exercise in Health and Disease*, W. B. Saunders Co., Philadelphia, 1990.

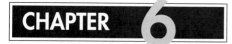

CHAPTER 6

IN THE GYM

OBJECTIVES

After reading this chapter, you should be able to do the following:

- Describe a variety of training programs, including circuit training, eccentric loading, and plyometric training.
- Demonstrate a proper lifting technique.
- Describe how to breathe properly during weight training.
- Understand how to spot correctly.

KEY TERMS

While reading this chapter, you will become familiar with the following terms:

- ► Circuit Training
- ► Eccentric Loading (or Negatives)
- ► Plyometric Exercises
- ► Sticking Points

BEFORE AND AFTER YOUR TRAINING PROGRAM

WARM-UP EXERCISES

The purpose of the warm-up period is to prepare the body for more vigorous activity and to reduce the chance of injury. A gradual warm-up period increases the blood flow to the muscles, which actually "warms" the muscles so they can function more effectively. The warm-up period should consist of a light aerobic period followed by flexibility exercises. The light aerobic period might consist of some light calisthenics, jogging in place, or five to ten minutes on stationary aerobic exercise equipment. Some suggested flexibility exercises are described in chapter 7. You can also warm up by lifting a light weight for ten to twelve repetitions. An adequate warm-up period should last at least ten minutes.

COOL-DOWN EXERCISES

The purpose of the cool-down period is to allow the body to gradually return to its pre-exercise resting state. The cool-down period basically consists of the same exercises as the warm-up period and should last between ten and fifteen minutes.

EXAMPLES OF DIFFERENT PROGRAMS

CIRCUIT TRAINING

Circuit training is a form of strength training that consists of a series of strength training exercises. It is an effective way of developing strength and flexibility, but has very little effect on aerobic endurance. A circuit training program has a series of eight to twelve exercise stations that the individual rapidly progresses through, spending a limited amount of time at each station. This is a popular form of training at many health clubs when time spent in the gym is limited, such as before or after work, or over the lunch hour. Best results are achieved if the entire circuit is completed three times.

ECCENTRIC LOADING

Remember that an eccentric contraction occurs when the muscle contracts and the muscle fibers lengthen. **Eccentric loading** (or performing **negatives**) allows you to develop strength while maintaining control of the weight. An example of performing a negative is to have a partner hand you a weight in the contracted position, and then you slowly return the weight to the starting position of the exer-

Example of a Circuit Training Workout	
Station 1	Hamstring and calf stretch
Station 2	Push-ups: 30 repetitions
Station 3	Rope skipping: 100 repetitions
Station 4	Bench press: 12 repetitions at 75% effort
Station 5	Triceps extensions: 8–12 repetitions each arm
Station 6	Bent-knee sit-ups: 25 repetitions
Station 7	Lateral pulldowns: 8–12 repetitions at 75% effort
Station 8	Biceps curls: 8–12 repetitions each arm

cise movement. Negatives are a popular and effective technique to develop strength and overcome **sticking points,** but they also seem to cause more fatigue and soreness than other methods.

PLYOMETRIC TRAINING

Plyometric training is a technique used to develop explosive strength and power. A **plyometric exercise** consists of a quick eccentric contraction followed by a powerful concentric contraction. The sudden stretch causes certain receptors in the muscles to stimulate a more powerful contraction. An example of a plyometric exercise is jumping off a bench, bending at the knees, and jumping back up onto the bench. Plyometric training is an effective method for improving muscular strength and endurance, but can cause injuries if not performed correctly.

LIFTING TECHNIQUE

GRIP

There are two common grips used in weight training, the overhand grip (knuckles up) and the underhand grip (palms up) (Figure 6-1). Both grips are appropriate for the specific exercise in question. For example, the overhand grip is commonly used to perform the lateral fly, shoulder press, etc., whereas the underhand grip is common for such lifts as the biceps curl. There are three common grip widths:

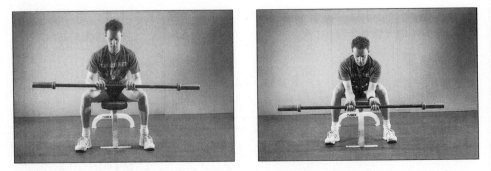

FIGURE 6-1 A. Overhand grip. **B.** Underhand grip.

normal, wide, and narrow. Most of the time the grip width should be approximately shoulder width apart. The most important things to consider with choosing a grip width are that it is comfortable and that you have a stable position to work from.

BREATHING

The golden rule regarding breathing during weight lifting is to inhale during the beginning of the lift and exhale as you complete the lift. Using the bench press as an example, once you have hold of the bar, you would inhale as you lower the bar toward your chest and exhale as you push the bar back to the starting position.

Never hold your breath during any part of a weight lifting movement. This can significantly increase your blood pressure and reduce the flow of oxygen to your brain, possibly causing you to pass out.

Fitness Tip

Normal, Wide, and Narrow Grips

Experiment with different grip widths and try to determine if changing the grip changes the body area stressed. Perform a bench press with a lighter weight than normal. Perform ten repetitions with a normal grip (a little more than shoulder width), narrow grip, and wide grip. Do you feel a difference? The narrow grip places greater stress on your triceps muscles, whereas the wide grip places greater stress on your shoulders and pectoral muscles. Try the same experiment with some other exercises and see what you find out.

General Lifting Technique

Most weight lifting injuries can be prevented if the proper technique is used.
- Always keep the weight close to your body.
- Lift with your legs.
- Avoid twisting when lifting.
- Lift the weight smoothly.
- Allow for adequate rest between sets.
- Never lift more than you are safely able to.
- Always use proper breathing.

REST

The amount of rest between workouts is just as important as the amount of time spent in workouts. Rest is needed between workouts to replace the energy stores in your muscles (glycogen) and to let your overall body systems recover from training. If you push too hard for too long, your body will eventually break down. Always take at least one day off between training sessions. In addition, always take at least one or two minutes to rest between exercise sets. Certain training systems recommend that you take as little time as possible between sets to get the most out of your training; however, this technique is not recommended for beginners.

COLLARS

There are a variety of collars in use today. Olympic bars typically have collars that screw on to hold the weight. Some gyms have quick release collars for use with regular and Olympic style bars. Some barbells have set amounts of weight on them, and the collars are permanently welded in place. All collars work well to keep the weight securely in place, as long as they are used. Some of the worst accidents have occurred from plates falling off a barbell during a lift. Just imagine what a 50 lb., 25 lb., or even 10 lb. plate would feel like falling on your toe. If collars are missing, or if there are not enough collars to go around, inform the management at once and do not begin lifting until they are secured on the bars you are using.

SPOTTING TECHNIQUE

The spotter's responsibility is to assist a partner in performing an exercise in a safe and effective manner. The first lesson a spotter needs to learn is to always

General Guidelines for Training with Weights

1. Always use collars on barbells and dumbbells.
2. Never perform one-repetition maximum lifts by yourself.
3. Always breathe out during the explosive part of the lift.
4. Always use proper form and technique.
5. Avoid fast or jerking motions. All lifting motions should be slow and controlled.
6. Keep weights as close to your body as possible.
7. Lift with your legs and keep your back straight when picking up a weight from the ground.
8. Rest between exercise sets.
9. Lift with individual goals in mind.

communicate with his/her partner. Before the lifter begins an exercise, the spotter should ask how many repetitions the lifter intends to do and if he/she is lifting a new amount of weight. The spotter should have a plan in mind if the lifter fails to lift the weight, and should always be alert and ready to grab the weight at any time (Figure 6-2). The spotter must be strong enough to lift the weight if the partner fails. Ideally, partners should be matched based on size and strength. As the partner performs the lift, the spotter should correct any problems with technique. Spotters should encourage and motivate their partners when training.

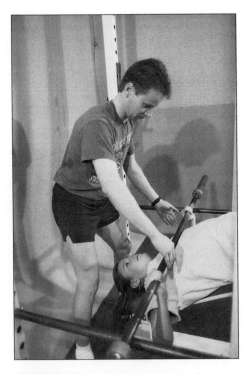

FIGURE 6-2 Correct spotting technique for decline bench press.

SUMMARY

- The warm-up period prepares the body for more vigorous activity and reduces the chance of injury.
- The cool-down period allows the body to gradually return to its pre-exercise state. It basically consists of the same exercises as the warm-up period.

- Circuit training is a form of strength training that consists of a series of strength training exercises. Circuit training is an effective way of developing strength and flexibility.
- Eccentric loading (performing negatives) is a technique that allows you to develop strength while maintaining control of the weight.
- Plyometric training is a technique used to develop explosive strength and power. A plyometric exercise consists of a quick eccentric contraction followed by a powerful concentric contraction.
- There are two common grips used in weight training: the overhand grip (knuckles up) and the underhand grip (palms up). There are also three common grip widths: normal, wide, and narrow. The grip width usually should be approximately shoulder width apart and should always be comfortable.
- The golden rule regarding breathing during weight lifting is to inhale during the beginning of the lift and exhale as you complete the lift.
- Rest is needed between workouts to replace the energy stores in your muscles (glycogen) and to let your overall body systems recover from training. In addition, always take at least one or two minutes to rest between exercise sets.
- All collars work well to keep the weight securely in place, as long as they are used.
- The spotter's responsibility is to assist a partner in performing an exercise in a safe and effective manner.

▶ **Circuit Training   p. 62**
A form of strength training that consists of a series of strength training exercises.

▶ **Eccentric Loading (or Negatives)   p. 62**
A technique that allows you to develop strength while maintaining control of the weight.

▶ **Plyometric Exercise   p. 63**
A technique that consists of a quick eccentric contraction followed by a powerful concentric contraction.

▶ **Sticking Points   p. 63**
The point in the range of motion of a weight training exercise that is the most difficult to move the weight through.

CHAPTER 7

THE **WARM-UP** ROUTINE

OBJECTIVES

After reading this chapter, you should be able to do the following:

- List the potential benefits and risks of stretching.
- Know the difference between the warm-up period and flexibility training.
- List several different warm-up routines.
- Understand the difference between static and dynamic stretching.
- List general flexibility training guidelines.
- Perform several upper and lower body stretches correctly.

KEY TERMS

While reading this chapter, you will become familiar with the following terms:

- ► Dynamic Stretching
- ► Flexibility
- ► Static Stretching
- ► Stretching
- ► Stretch Reflex
- ► Warm-Up Period

WARM-UP REVISITED

As mentioned in chapter 6, the **warm-up period** is an integral part of the overall exercise session. The warm-up period occurs before the actual exercise session begins. Many people believe the warm-up period should consist of **stretching** only, but there is more to the warm-up period than this. There are three primary benefits of warming up prior to exercise: physiological, psychological, and injury prevention. Warming up prior to exercise increases blood flow to the working muscles and gradually increases the temperature of the muscles, both of which better prepare the body for exercise. The warm-up period can increase adrenaline, making one more "psyched-up" to exercise. And lastly, warming up before exercise can reduce the stress on the heart and possibly reduce the chance of musculoskeletal injuries as well. The following Fitness Tip provides a few practical guidelines.

Many of the benefits to be obtained from a good warm-up routine cannot be achieved solely by stretching. In fact, performing stretching exercises prior to a good warm-up routine may actually increase the risk of injury. Thus, the correct way to warm up is to do some gradual aerobic exercise, such as walking, running in place, stationary cycling, etc., for five to ten minutes, and then, if you want, perform some stretching exercises. Stretching exercise solely intended to improve flexibility may also be performed following the exercise session.

FLEXIBILITY TRAINING

Stretching is commonly referred to as flexibility training. **Flexibility** is defined as the range of motion in a given joint or combination of joints. Flexibility training is an important part of a balanced fitness program but is often overlooked, even by experienced athletes. Flexibility training is often viewed as unnecessary and

Fitness Tip

Selected Warm-Up Routines

Identical to Performance: Performing the bench press at 50 to 65 percent of maximal weight for one to two sets. Such routines can also be perfomed with any exercise.

Directly Related to Perfomance: Performing squats with the barbell, but no weights. This is a great way to warm up prior to specific lifts.

Indirectly Related to Performance: Five to ten minutes of stationary cycling, followed by some stretching. This is a more general warm-up routine.

time-consuming. Although scientific evidence demonstrating the benefits of flexibility training is limited, it is generally agreed among most medical experts that flexibility training is important for optimal health and peak athletic performance.

Flexibility training is used to improve performance and reduce the possibility of injury, and in sports medicine fields (physical therapy) as a component of injury treatment and rehabilitation. It is well known that a decrease in flexibility is inevitable with age and physical inactivity. One of the most common ailments for adults, chronic low back pain, is primarily due to a decrease in flexibility, along with inadequate strength. Some sports require movement patterns that demand a great deal of flexibility—for example, the butterfly stroke in swimming. The importance of superior flexibility in sports such as basketball or football is debatable. Regardless, adequate flexibility should help reduce muscle tension, improve posture and coordination, reduce body stiffness, possibly reduce injury, and enhance athletic performance. The potential benefits of stretching include: (1) increased performance, (2) increased joint stability, (3) increased joint range of motion, (4) enhanced warm-up results, (5) injury prevention, and (6) decreased recovery time.

There are some potential risks associated with stretching. Attention has recently been focused on the timing of stretching. Current theory suggests that stretching be performed after a brief warm-up period. The logic behind such practice is based on the fact that preliminary movement raises the temperature of connective tissue, causing collagen to become softer and more elastic. An increased potential for injury is possible if stretching is performed prior to an active warm-up. The risk of injury from stretching is greatest when performed by poorly conditioned individuals or individuals with a pre-existing injury, and when stretches are performed with poor technique.

STRETCHING TECHNIQUE

Static stretching involves stretching the muscle and connective tissue of the joint passively to the extreme range of the joint. Static stretching is safer and more effective than dynamic stretching. **Dynamic stretching** involves repeated, bouncing movements that stretch the muscles (e.g., repeatedly bouncing forward to touch your toes). This type of stretching is not as effective as static stretching and can lead to increased injury because it stimulates the stretch reflex. When a muscle is stretched too fast, specialized receptors in the muscle called muscle spindles stimulate the muscle to contract so that it is not overstretched. This phenomenon is referred to as the **stretch reflex**. Static stretching does not stimulate the stretch reflex, whereas dynamic stretching does.

Static stretching exercises should be performed after a mild warm-up period to increase the temperature of the muscles and connective tissue. The static stretch should be held for ten to fifteen seconds. During the performance of a static stretch, the position should always be held just below the threshold for pain. Static stretching causes gradual inhibition of muscle spindle activation, which allows for greater long-term range of motion maintenance. Perform each of the stretches listed below following a brief warm-up period.

Fitness Tip

General Flexibility Training Guidelines

- Warm up for a few minutes prior to stretching.
- The static stretch should be held for about ten to fifteen seconds.
- During the performance of a static stretch, the position should always be held just below the threshold for pain.
- Move slowly from one position to the next.
- Stretching exercises can be performed before exercise, following a brief warm-up, and following exercise.
- To improve overall flexibility, upper and lower body stretches should be performed on a regular basis.
- If a particular stretch causes pain or discomfort, avoid it or seek advice from a health and fitness professional to determine if you are performing the stretch correctly.

STRETCHING EXERCISES

Does everyone need to stretch before training? How much flexibility is good? The answers to these questions are not known. The fact is, most people feel they benefit from some simple stretching before exercise. Do you need to perform all of the stretches before lifting? The answer is no. Listed below are some commonly performed stretches individuals use in the weight room prior to lifting. Select a range of stretches that will benefit your individual lifting program or consult a trainer to help you put together a stretching routine that will give you the best results.

STRETCH #1: HEEL PULL

Brace yourself against a solid object with one hand. With the opposite hand, grasp the top of your foot and slowly pull it toward your buttocks. Repeat with the opposite leg (Figure 7-1).

STRETCH #2: CALF STRETCH

Stand approximately 1 to 2 feet away from a wall or tree. Move one foot in close to the tree while keeping the back leg straight behind you with the foot and heel flat on the ground. Slowly move your hips forward, keeping your back foot on the ground. You should feel a slight stretch in your calf muscles. Repeat with the opposite leg (Figure 7-2).

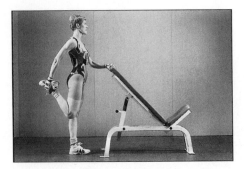

FIGURE 7-1 Heel pull.

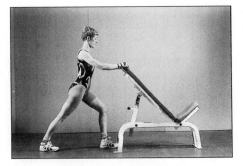

FIGURE 7-2 Calf stretch.

STRETCH #3: HAMSTRING STRETCH

Rest one of your legs on an object 2 to 3 feet high. Keep the leg that is on the object straight, and slowly bend forward. You should feel a slight stretch in your hamstring muscles. Repeat with the opposite leg.

STRETCH #4: LUNGE

Place your right foot about 12 to 18 inches in front of your left foot. Tuck your buttocks tightly under your hips while contracting your abdominal muscles. You should feel the stretch in the front of the hip region of the rear leg. Repeat with the opposite leg (Figure 7-3).

STRETCH #5: LOW BACK STRETCH

Lay on your back and pull both knees into the torso until a sufficient stretch is achieved in the low back. In all stretches it is important to go only to the point where the athlete feels the stretch, but is not in pain (Figure 7-4).

STRETCH #6: SUPINE HAMSTRING STRETCH

Lay on your back and pull one leg up to a stretched position. The leg should remain as straight as possible. The opposite leg is bent with the heel on the floor. Alternate legs (Figure 7-5).

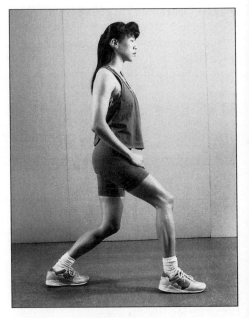

FIGURE 7-3 Lunge.

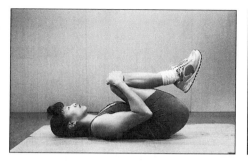

FIGURE 7-4 Low back stretch.

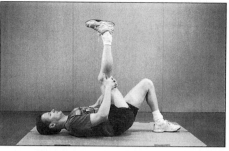

FIGURE 7-5 Supine hamstring stretch.

STRETCH #7: MODIFIED HURDLER'S STRETCH

Sit on the floor with one leg extended and the other leg bent and turned outward (heel against the thigh of the straight leg). Bend forward at the waist (leaning toward the straight leg) until a stretch is achieved and then hold this position for the required count. Alternate legs (Figure 7-6).

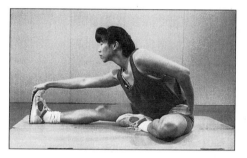

FIGURE 7-6 Modified hurdler's stretch.

STRETCH #8: TRICEPS STRETCH

Take one elbow and pull the arm behind the head and down until a stretch is felt in the back of the arm. Hold for the desired count. Repeat with the opposite arm (Figure 7-7).

STRETCH #9: SHOULDER AND CHEST STRETCH

Place one arm parallel to the floor and back behind the torso. You can hold on to a wall, a partner, or whatever is available. To further improve the effectiveness of this stretch, try turning away from the side being stretched until the stretch is felt in the shoulder and lateral chest region. Alternate sides (Figure 7-8).

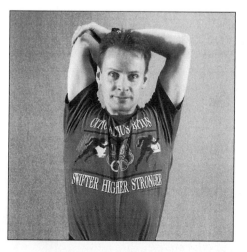

FIGURE 7-7 Triceps stretch.

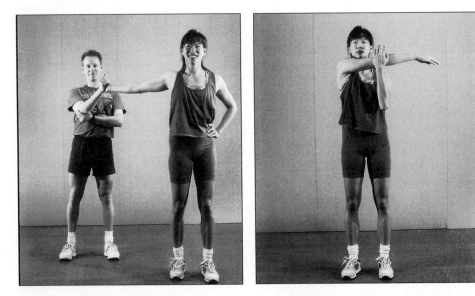

FIGURE 7-8 Shoulder and chest stretch.   **FIGURE 7-9** Rotator cuff stretch.

STRETCH #10: ROTATOR CUFF STRETCH

Grasp the elbow of the opposite arm (keeping it bent at a 90 degree angle) and pull it across the chest until the stretch is felt. Alternate arms (Figure 7-9).

SUMMARY

- The warm-up period is an integral part of the overall exercise session.
- There are three primary benefits of warming up: physiological (increased blood flow to the working muscles and a gradual increase in the temperature of the muscles), psychological (increased adrenaline), and injury prevention (reduced stress on the heart prior to exercise and reduced risk of musculoskeletal injuries).
- Warm-up routines can be identical to performance, directly related to performance, or indirectly related to performance.
- Stretching prior to a good warm-up routine may actually increase the risk of injury.
- Flexibility is defined as the range of motion in a given joint or combination of joints. Flexibility training is an important part of a balanced fitness program but is often overlooked, even by experienced athletes.
- Adequate flexibility should help reduce muscle tension, improve posture and coordination, reduce body stiffness, possibly reduce injury, and enhance athletic performance.

- The potential benefits of stretching include: (1) increased performance, (2) increased joint stability, (3) increased joint range of motion, (4) enhanced warm-up results, (5) injury prevention, and (6) decreased recovery time.
- The risk of injury from stretching is greatest when performed by poorly conditioned individuals or individuals with a preexisting injury, and when stretches are performed with poor technique.
- Static stretching is perhaps the safest and most effective form of stretching.
- Dynamic stretching can lead to increased injury because it stimulates the stretch reflex.
- When muscles are stretched too fast, the stretch reflex is stimulated to invoke the muscle to contract in order to prevent potential injury.
- Static stretching exercises should be performed after a mild warm-up period. Static stretches should be held for about ten to fifteen seconds. During the performance of a static stretch, the position should always be held just below the threshold for pain.

► **Dynamic Stretching   p. 70**
Stretching that involves uncontrolled or bouncing movements.

► **Flexibility   p. 69**
The range of motion in a given joint or combination of joints.

► **Static Stretching   p. 70**
Stretching the muscles and connective tissue of the joint passively to the extreme range of the joint.

► **Stretching   p. 69**
A series of exercise movements that lead to improved flexibility.

► **Stretch Reflex   p. 70**
A protective mechanism that occurs when muscles are stretched rapidly (during dynamic stretching) that results in a reflex contraction.

► **Warm-Up Period   p. 69**
The period prior to an exercise session that involves activities that prepare the body for exercise.

Assessment 7-1

Determining Your Low Back and Hamstring Flexibility

Name _____   Section _____   Date _____

One of the most common health ailments for adults is chronic low back pain. Poor low back and hamstring flexibility have been linked to chronic low back pain. The trunk flexion (sit and reach) test is a simple and economical test for evaluating your low back and hamstring flexibility.

1. Before starting this test make sure you have properly warmed up to begin exercise.
2. Remove your shoes and sit on the floor with your legs together, knees flat on the floor, and feet flat against a vertical surface.
3. Bend forward at the waist and reach as far forward as possible with the fingers (Figure 7-10).
4. Scoring is determined by measuring the distance, in inches, you can reach either in front of or beyond the vertical surface. Use Table 7-1 to evaluate your score.

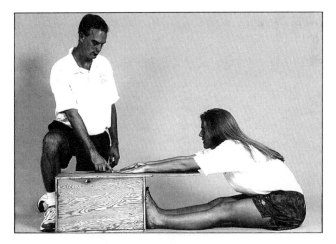

FIGURE 7-10 Feet are flat against the box with legs straight and head held up.

TABLE 7-1
Scoring Your Low Back and Hamstring Flexibility Test

Classification	Women	Men
Excellent	8″	7″
Good	5–7″	4–6″
Average	2–4″	1–3″
Poor	0″	0″

Scoring data from Prentice, *Fitness for College and Life*, 5e, 1997, Mosby-Year Book Inc., St. Louis.

Assessment 7-2

SHOULDER FLEXION

Name   Section   Date

1. Before starting this test, make sure you have properly warmed up for exercise.
2. Lie facedown on the floor with your arms fully extended overhead, chin touching the floor.
3. Grab a straight edge (yardstick or wooden rod) and hold it with your hands shoulder width apart.
4. Try to raise the stick as high as possible while keeping your chin on the floor (Figure 7-11).
5. Scoring is determined by how high you can raise the straight edge off the ground. Use Table 7-2 to evaluate your score. (See table on page 80.)

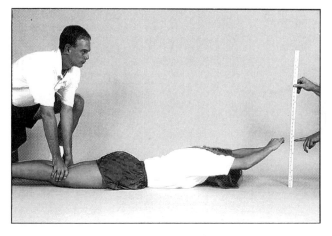

FIGURE 7-11 It may help to have someone hold your legs while a third person measures the results.

80 WEIGHT TRAINING

TABLE 7-2
Scoring Your Shoulder Flexion Test

Classification	Women	Men
Excellent	27″	26″
Good	24–26″	23–25″
Average	21–23″	20–22″
Poor	0–20″	0–19″

Scoring data from Prentice, *Fitness for College and Life*, 5e, 1997, Mosby-Year Book Inc., St. Louis.

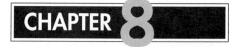

CHAPTER 8

ARM EXERCISES

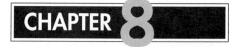

OBJECTIVES

After reading this chapter, you should be able to do the following:

- Identify the muscles of the upper arm and cite their primary functions.
- Identify the major muscles of the lower arm and cite their functions.
- Know how to perform several exercises for each of the previously identified muscles.

KEY TERMS

While reading this chapter, you will become familiar with the following terms:

► Anconeus
► Biceps Brachii
► Brachialis
► Extensor Carpi Radialis
► Extensor Carpi Ulnaris
► Flexor Carpi Radialis
► Flexor Carpi Ulnaris

► Pronator Quadratus
► Pronator Teres
► Supinator
► Triceps Brachii

Arms are the first area most people think about when they consider weight training. Most people flex their biceps brachii when someone asks to see their muscles. With arms it is important (and with the total body as well) to stress balanced development of the muscles in question. In other words, if you're working the biceps don't skip the triceps. If you're working the forearm flexors don't skip the forearm extensors. Increasing arm strength can help with the performance of many common tasks such as carrying groceries, maintenance around the house, and improving sports-specific performance. Working on your forearm flexors and extensors can have a significant impact on your tennis and golf games. So let's get started! Understanding muscle function will enable you to have a better handle on which exercises will work best for your specific program.

EXERCISES FOR THE TRICEPS

TRICEPS EXTENSION

Muscles Used: **Triceps brachii, anconeus**
Exercise Technique: Lay down on a bench with your feet up on the bench for back support. Take a fairly narrow grip (6 to 12 inches between hands) on the bar, using an EZ curl bar if possible. Lower the bar to just above your forehead and then, keeping elbows stationary, lift the bar by extending the lower arms. Performing this exercise on a decline bench will stress the lateral and medial head as well as the long head of the triceps (Figure 8-1).

MACHINE TRICEPS EXTENSION

Muscles Used: Triceps, anconeus
Exercise Technique: For this exercise, start seated in the upright position. When your elbows are on the pads, they should be in a straight line with your shoulder joint. Grasp the handles with your thumbs facing your torso, the long pivot arm of the bar should be facing you as well. Press the handles away from yourself, using only your extensors. Keep the elbows in contact with the pads at all times.

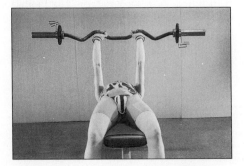 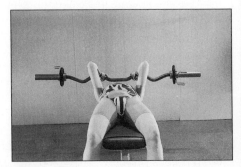

FIGURE 8-1 Triceps extension.

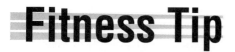
Fitness Tip

Spotting the Triceps Extension

When spotting the triceps extension the spotter should be positioned directly behind the lifter and help the bar upward with gentle assistance if needed. Always be ready to take the bar from the lifter when the fatigue point is reached.

CLOSE-GRIP BENCH PRESS

Muscles Used: Triceps, anconeus, anterior deltoid, pectoralis major
Exercise Technique: The lifter begins in the same position as that used in the triceps extension. The hand spacing is also identical. The lifter is handed the bar or takes it off the bench and lowers it to chest level. The elbows are allowed to flare out on this exercise. When the bar reaches the chest, the direction is reversed and the bar is pressed out to complete extension. Spotting is the same as in the triceps extension (Figure 8-2).

DUMBBELL KICKBACKS

Muscles Used: Triceps (medial and lateral heads in particular), anconeus
Exercise Technique: This exercise may be done standing while leaning forward and bracing on the knee, or kneeling on a bench. The lift begins with the elbow of the arm holding the dumbbell at 90 degrees. The arm is then extended while the elbow remains motionless and close to the body (Figure 8-3).

ONE-ARM FRENCH CURL

Muscles Used: Triceps, anconeus
Exercise Technique: Begin in either the seated or standing position. Hold a dumbbell above your head with your fist thumb down (and away from the head). The opposite arm may be used to brace the exercising arm at the elbow area. From the extended position, lower the arm until a good stretch is felt on the triceps muscle. At this point raise the arm once again to the starting position (Figure 8-4).

TRICEPS PRESSDOWN

Muscles Used: Triceps, anconeus
Exercise Technique: Begin by facing the W-shaped or inverted V-shaped bar used in triceps pressdowns. Grasp the bar with a narrow grip (4 to 6 inches apart) with palms facing away from you. The bar at this point should be at chest height

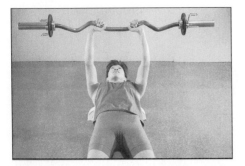 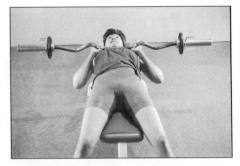

FIGURE 8-2 Close-grip bench press.

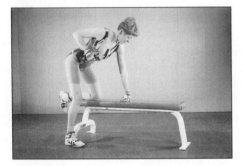 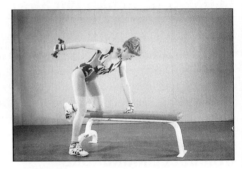

FIGURE 8-3 Dumbbell kickback.

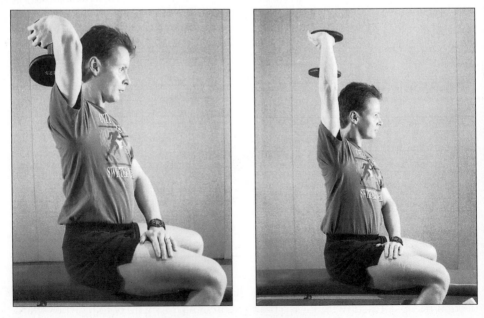

FIGURE 8-4 One-arm French curl.

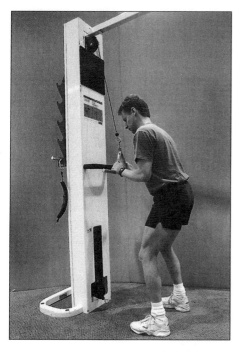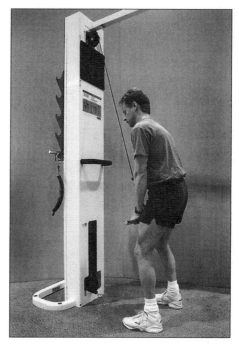

FIGURE 8-5 Triceps pressdown.

and your elbows should be pressed into the side of the torso. Push the bar down until the arms are completely extended. When returning the bar to the starting position keep the elbows at the side and actively resist the bar's upward motion. Using the rope as a handle on this exercise stresses the medial head in addition to the long and lateral heads of the triceps brachii (Figure 8-5).

EXERCISES FOR THE BICEPS

PREACHER CURL

Muscles Used: **Biceps brachii, brachialis**
Exercise Technique: This exercise is most efficient when done with a preacher curl bench. With this device it is possible to sit down and with arms extended and palms up, grasp the bar with a shoulder width grip (the entire upper arm should be placed firmly against the pad). From this position, the elbow is flexed and the bar is brought upward to chin level (Figure 8-6).

DUMBBELL CURL

Muscles Used: Biceps (greatest emphasis on the medial head), brachialis
Exercise Technique: This exercise may be done seated or standing. Begin with dumbbells held in each hand, wrists supinated and arms extended. At this point

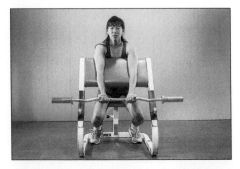
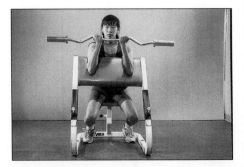

FIGURE 8-6 Preacher curl.

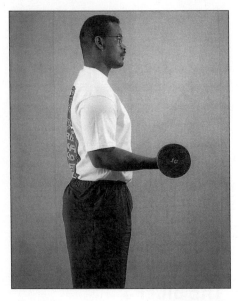
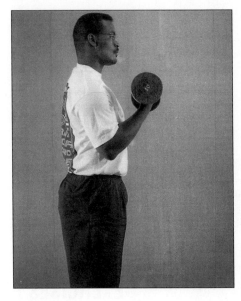

FIGURE 8-7 Dumbbell curl.

the arms may be flexed unilaterally (one at a time) or bilaterally to the complete contraction phase. This exercise should not involve swaying of the torso or legs or assistance from any other muscle group. A barbell may be substituted for dumbbells in a variant of this exercise called the EZ curl (Figure 8-7).

SEATED MACHINE CURL

Muscles Used: Biceps, brachialis

Exercise Technique: Before beginning this exercise be certain that your elbows (which are placed on the pads in front of the torso) are in line with the shoulder joint. Then simply grasp the handles with your palms facing upward. Start in the extended, but not hyperextended, position. From this point, pull the handles toward yourself until a complete contraction is achieved.

Fitness Tip

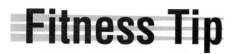

Spotting the Standing Curl

When spotting the standing curl with a barbell, the spotter should stand directly in front of the lifter. The spotter should assist the lifter by placing his palms up (inside of the hands of the lifter) and exerting force upward as needed.

CONCENTRATION CURL

Muscles Used: Biceps, brachialis
Exercise Technique: This exercise is performed seated with the dumbbell held palm upward and the elbow against the inside of the knee. From the position where the forearm is extended, the weight is curled up toward the torso while the elbow remains motionless (Figure 8-8).

EXERCISES FOR THE FOREARMS

WRIST CURL

Muscles Used: **Flexor carpi ulnaris, flexor carpi radialis**
Exercise Technique: This exercise is performed while seated on a bench. The bar is gripped with hands approximately 6 inches apart and palms upward. Let about

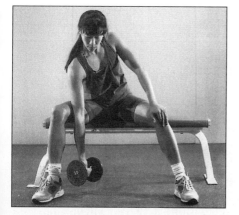
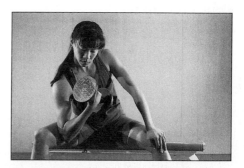

FIGURE 8-8 Concentration curl.

3 or 4 inches of the forearm hang over the bench while holding the bar. Bracing the forearms against the inside of the knees may be helpful. Raise the weight by curling the palms toward the forearm and then reversing direction. Do not open the hands and roll the bar onto the fingers (Figure 8-9).

WRIST EXTENSION

Muscles Used: **Extensor carpi ulnaris, extensor carpi radialis**

Exercise Technique: This exercise is also performed while seated on a bench. Grip the bar slightly wider than shoulder width with the palms facing down. Again you should have 3 to 4 inches of your forearm over the edge of your knee. The movement starts with the weight down and the wrists flexed, and ends with the weight up and the wrists fully extended (Figure 8-10).

REVERSE CURL

Muscles Used: Brachialis

Exercise Technique: While standing, grip the bar with hands shoulder width apart and palms facing away from the body. Rest the bar on the thighs. Lift the weight by curling the arms toward the chest until complete contraction is reached. Keep the elbows stationary (Figure 8-11).

WRIST PRONATION AND SUPINATION

Muscles Used: **Pronator quadratus, pronator teres, supinator**

Exercise Technique: This exercise is performed using a dumbbell loaded on one end only. While seated, grasp the dumbbell with one arm at a 90 degree angle, leaving approximately 4 inches of the forearm over the bench. The other arm shoud be placed firmly on the bench just behind the elbow to stabilize the

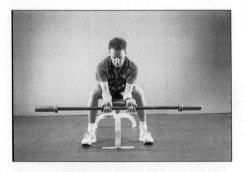

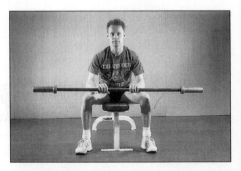

FIGURE 8-9 Wrist curl.   **FIGURE 8-10** Wrist extension.

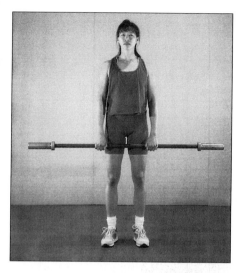 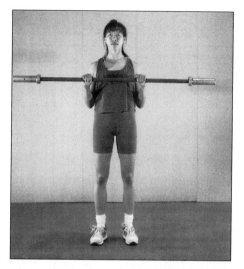

FIGURE 8-11 Reverse curl.

exercising arm. The dumbbell is then rotated from a palm-down (pronation) to a palm-up (supination) position while the elbow remains stationary. Control the movement, do not simply let the wrist drop from side to side (Figure 8-12).

▶ **Anconeus   p. 82**
Action: forearm extensor.

▶ **Biceps Brachii   p. 85**
Action: flexes elbow joint and supinates (turns hand over to the palm-up position) the forearm.

▶ **Brachialis   p. 85**
Action: forearm flexion.

▶ **Extensor Carpi Radialis   p. 88**
Action: wrist extension.

▶ **Extensor Carpi Ulnaris   p. 88**
Action: wrist extension.

▶ **Flexor Carpi Radialis   p. 87**
Action: wrist flexion and hand abduction.

▶ **Flexor Carpi Ulnaris   p. 87**
Action: wrist flexion and hand adduction.

▶ **Pronator Quadratus   p. 88**
Action: pronates the forearm.

▶ **Pronator Teres   p. 88**
Action: pronates the forearm.

▶ **Supinator   p. 88**
Action: assists the biceps brachii in supinating the forearm.

▶ **Triceps Brachii   p. 82**
Action: forearm extensor.

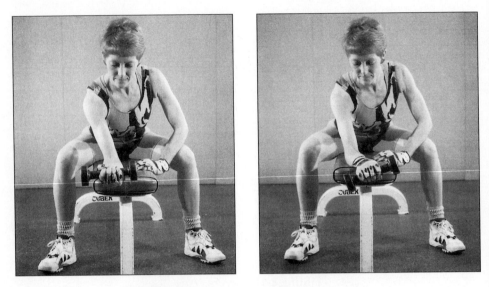

FIGURE 8-12 Wrist pronation and supination.

SUMMARY

- Triceps brachii and the anconeus are upper arm forearm extensors.
- Biceps brachii and the brachialis are two of the major upper arm muscles that perform forearm flexion.
- Wrist flexors include the flexor carpi ulnaris and flexor carpi radialis.
- Wrist extensors include the extensor carpi ulnaris and extensor carpi radialis.
- Pronation and supination in the forearm are caused by the following muscles respectively: pronator quadratus, pronator teres, and the supinator.
- Exercises for working the arm musculature include the following: triceps extension, machine triceps extension, close-grip bench press, dumbbell kickback, one-arm French curl, triceps pressdown, preacher curl, dumbbell curl, seated machine curl, concentration curl, wrist curl, wrist extension, reverse curl, and wrist pronation and supination.
- Pick and choose from the above list to match your program needs. Do not do more than two exercises per body part per session unless you are attempting to train for bodybuilding purposes.

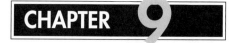
CHEST **EXERCISES**

OBJECTIVES

After reading this chapter, you should be able to do the following:

- Identify the muscles of the chest area and cite their primary functions.
- Know several exercises for each of the previously listed muscles.

KEY TERMS

While reading this chapter, you will become familiar with the following terms:

- ► Coracobrachialis
- ► Horizontal Adduction
- ► Pectoralis Major
- ► Serratus Anterior

Having a shapely, well-defined chest is highly valued by our culture. To verify this statement, one need only pick up a fashion or fitness magazine to find a veritable cornucopia of exercises, fashions, and other assorted advice to highlight, improve, or hide (if this is a weak area for the reader) this section of your physique. Beyond the obvious aesthetic appeal of strong and shapely chest muscles lies their inherent value. A strong chest can help in activities as varied as bringing in the groceries to waxing the car, so let's work those pecs!

EXERCISES FOR THE CHEST

BENCH PRESS

Muscles Used: **Pectoralis major,** anterior deltoid, triceps brachii, **serratus anterior**

Exercise Technique: Begin by lying with the back on a flat bench apparatus. Normally a shoulder width grip is used, although variations on width are possible. Wider grips place more stress on the pectoralis major, while narrower grips place more stress on the triceps brachii. Begin the exercise with the arms extended and the weight held overhead. Lower the bar with control to the chest area, stopping at or slightly below the nipple line. After a brief pause, drive the bar back up to the extended position. Do not arch the back or leave the bench with your hips when bench pressing. A false grip with thumbs behind the bar is not recommended, as this can lead to dropping the bar very quickly onto oneself. Spotters are a necessity in this lift and all its variations (Figure 9-1).

INCLINE BENCH PRESS

Muscles Used: Pectoralis major (emphasis on sternal portion), anterior deltoid, triceps brachii

Exercise Technique: This exercise is performed while supine on a 45 degree incline bench. Lower the bar from the extended position to the upper chest area, approximately midway between the clavicles and the nipple line. Then, press the bar upward to the extended position at an angle that is in line with the bench supports. Do not allow the bar to travel out and away from the body (Figure 9-2).

SEATED CHEST PRESS

Muscles Used: Pectoralis major, anterior deltoid, triceps brachii, serratus anterior

Exercise Technique: Most upright chest press stations have horizontal and vertical handles. With the horizontal handles the lifter keeps the palms down and the

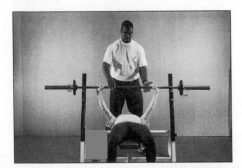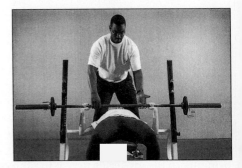

FIGURE 9-1 Flat bench press.

Fitness Tip

Spotting the Bench Press

The bench press is one of the most common lifts on which a spotter's assistance might be needed. However, it is often spotted incorrectly. Do not attempt to spot this lift with a palms-up (curling grip) position. This is the weakest position for spotting, and if someone truly fails in the bench press most spotters would have a difficult time lifting the weight off of the lifter in this manner. The most effective way to spot (see figure 9-1) is with a mixed grip. The strong hand should be facing palm down and the weaker hand should face palm up. This is the same grip used in the dead-lift. It is the strongest grip position and it allows you to lift with your legs and shoulder muscles, not just your arms. Always pay attention when you are spotting. The lifter could fail in a split second and if you are looking away, the bar will be on his face or throat before you react.

elbows up. When the vertical handle option (which focuses more on the triceps as opposed to the horizontal handle) is chosen, the hands are in the neutral or thumbs-up position and the elbows are in and next to the torso. After the weight is chosen and the seat is adjusted so that your chest is in alignment with the handles, simply push the handles away from the torso, lower, and repeat. There is no weight to become pinned under, but you must still keep your back flat against the pad. Back strain is a possibility if you arch in an attempt to push too much weight (Figure 9-3.)

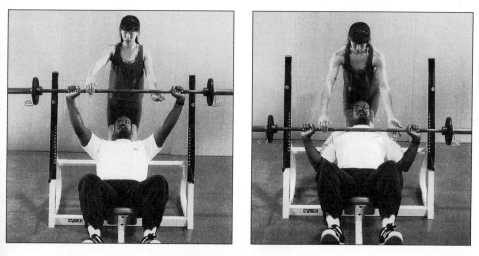

FIGURE 9-2 Incline bench press.

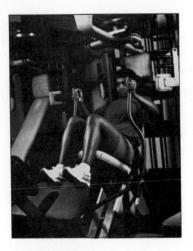

FIGURE 9-3 Seated chest press.

DECLINE BENCH PRESS

Muscles Used: Pectoralis major (lower or distal portion of the muscle), anterior deltoid, triceps brachii

Exercise Technique: On a decline bench set approximately at a 30 degree angle, lie in the supine position with feet hooked under the pads at the far end of the bench. From the extended position, lower the bar to the lower part of the chest, just below the nipple line. Then press the bar straight up toward the uprights. In this and all bench press variations, dumbbells may be substituted for the barbell. This option gives a slightly greater range of motion and allows the individual to work each side independently (Figure 9-4).

DUMBBELL FLY

Muscles Used: Pectoralis major, anterior deltoid, serratus anterior

Exercise Technique: Begin by lying supine on a flat or incline bench with a dumbbell in each hand. The palms are facing each other with arms extended and bent at a 90 degree angle. The dumbbells are above the sternum. Lower the dumbbells to the point of a comfortable stretch at the bottom position and then return

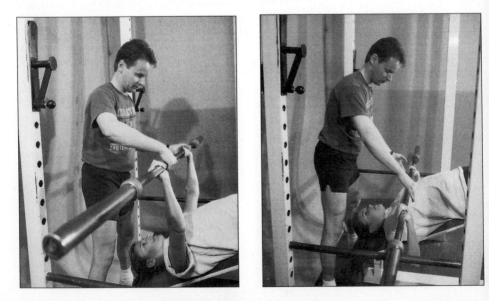

FIGURE 9-4 Decline bench press.

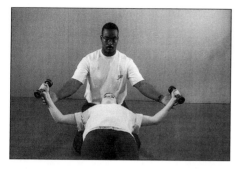 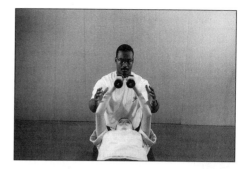

FIGURE 9-5 Dumbbell fly.

them to the starting position. A useful mental image for this exercise is to imagine hugging a tree or barrel to facilitate keeping the arms wide (Figure 9-5).

CABLE CROSSOVER

Muscles Used: Pectoralis major, anterior deltoid, biceps brachii, **coracobrachialis**
Exercise Technique: Stand inside a cable crossover machine and grasp one handle in each hand. The handles should be at or slightly above ear height. Position yourself with the torso inclined forward at approximately a 10 to 30 degree angle and place one leg ahead of the body for stability. Begin with the arms extended out to the sides, but with a slight bend at the elbow. Pull the handles into the midline of the chest until the forearms cross, making an X position. If you do not have a cable crossover station, some gyms will have a fly or pec-dec machine. If neither of these options are available, substitute with the dumbbell fly (Figure 9-6).

DIPS

Muscles Used: Pectoralis major, triceps, trapezius, deltoid

Fitness Tip

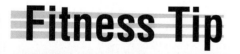

Spotting the Dumbbell Fly

When spotting this move, you should be low to the ground and directly behind the lifter. Place your hands on the lifter's wrists and go with each movement. Lift upward as needed. This helps to prevent the lifter from losing the dumbbells in a weak position.

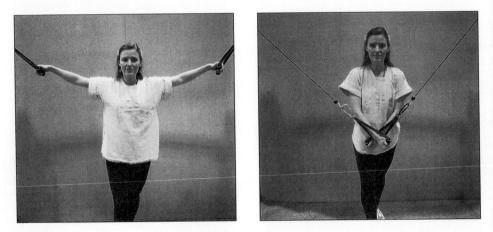

FIGURE 9-6 Cable crossover.

Exercise Technique: To start, brace the body on the dipping bars with arms locked. Ideally the bars should be adjusted to be no farther apart than the distance between your elbow and middle fingertip. Lower the body in a controlled fashion until a 90 degree angle is reached at the elbow and then push up again (without kicking or swinging) to the extended position. Keeping the torso upright puts most of the stress on the triceps; leaning into the movement puts more stress on the pectorals. If you have difficulty doing the concentric or upward phase of this movement, try jumping up and then slowly lowering yourself down. Eventually you will have the strength to do the concentric phase of the movement. This exercise places a significant amount of stress on the shoulder joint, therefore use caution if this is a problem area (Figure 9-7).

Fitness Tip

Work for a Balance

Important note! Do not make the mistake of so many weight trainers in the field today. Always work for balance in muscle groups. Agonist (prime movers) muscles or muscle groups should always be in balance with antagonist (opposite of prime movers) muscles or muscle groups. If you are going to work your pecs and chest musculature, be certain to balance this out with an equal amount of back work. Remember the back should be a stronger muscle group area anyway.

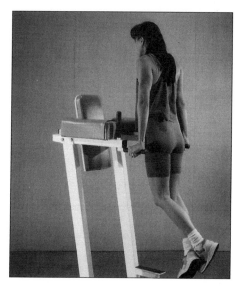 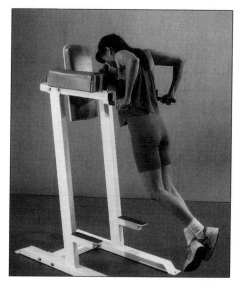

FIGURE 9-7 Dip.

SUMMARY

- The pectoralis major is responsible for drawing the scapula forward and downward, as well as **horizontal adduction** of the arm.
- The serratus anterior protracts and holds the scapula against the chest wall and it also causes horizontal adduction of the arm.
- The coracobrachialis causes flexion and adduction of the humerus.
- Exercises for working the chest musculature include the following: flat bench press, incline bench press, seated chest press, decline bench press, dumbbell fly, cable crossover, pec-dec, machine fly, and dip.

▶ **Coracobrachialis   p. 95**
Action: flexion and adduction of the humerus.

▶ **Horizontal Adduction   p. 97**
Moving the shoulder joint in toward the front of the body with the arm parallel to the floor.

▶ **Pectoralis Major   p. 92**
Action: draws scapula forward and downward.

▶ **Serratus Anterior   p. 92**
Action: protracts and holds scapula against chest wall, horizontal adduction of the arm.

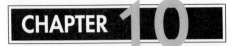

CHAPTER 10

UPPER BACK AND SHOULDER EXERCISES

OBJECTIVES

After reading this chapter, you should be able to do the following:

- Identify the major muscles of the upper back and cite their primary functions.
- Identify the major muscles of the shoulder area and cite their primary functions.
- Know several exercises for each of the previously listed muscles.

KEY TERMS

While reading this chapter, you will become familiar with the following terms:

- ▶ Deltoid
- ▶ Infraspinatus
- ▶ Subscapularis
- ▶ Supraspinatus
- ▶ Teres Minor
- ▶ Trapezius

Traditionally, a broad and muscular upper back and shoulder area has always been associated with serious weight lifters and bodybuilders. This is not to say that the average male or female would not appreciate a healthy and fit-looking upper back and shoulder area. On the contrary, many fashions are tailored to accentuate these areas, and therefore fit and toned muscles will only serve to highlight one's appearance. No weight trained man or woman will ever need shoulder pads! Strength in these areas will also aid in good posture and in slowing the onset of fatigue from a long day at the desk or in the office. With these thoughts in mind, let's look at some exercises designed to improve your shoulders and upper back.

UPPER BACK AND SHOULDER EXERCISES

UPRIGHT ROW

Muscles Used: **Trapezius, deltoid,** biceps
Exercise Technique: This exercise is performed standing with a grip of approximately 6 to 12 inches between hands. The palms are facing the torso and the feet are shoulder width apart. Begin with the barbell just above the knees and the arms extended. Pull the barbell up to clavicle or chin level. Keep the back straight and lead with the elbows. This exercise may also be performed with a dumbbell in each hand (Figure 10-1).

SHRUG

Muscles Used: Trapezius
Exercise Technique: The starting position for this exercise is identical to that of the upright row except that a shoulder width grip is used on the bar. Begin with the arms extended and finish with the trapezius muscle being shrugged as high as possible. The arms remain straight throughout the exercise and other muscle group involvement should be minimized (Figure 10-2).

SHOULDER PRESS

Muscles Used: Deltoid, triceps, pectoralis major
Exercise Technique: This exercise may be done seated or standing, with dumbbells or a barbell. A belt should be worn and a spotter is needed for both variations. Start with the barbell on the front of the upper chest area, with the hands shoulder width apart and palms facing outward. Press the barbell up evenly to complete extension without arching the back. A variation of this exercise is the press behind the neck, in which the barbell starts behind the neck and is pressed upward. This variation

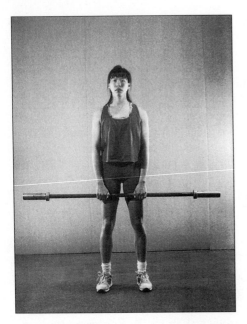
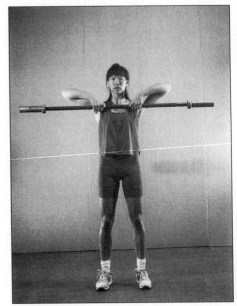

FIGURE 10-1 Upright row.

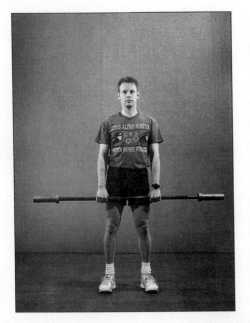
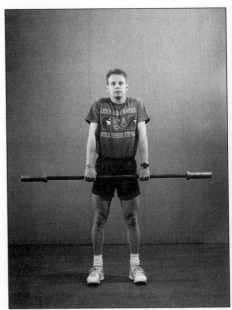

FIGURE 10-2 Shrug.

stimulates the trapezius in addition to deltoid and triceps involvement (Figure 10-3).

SMITH MACHINE SHOULDER PRESS

Muscles Used: Deltoid, triceps, pectoralis major

Exercise Technique: This exercise variant employs the commonly found Smith machine and is a very safe substitute for the regular seated or standing press. First, set up a bench inside the machine with the seat at a 90 degree angle. At this point assume a shoulder width or slightly wider grip on the bar, with the back pressed firmly against the upright bench. The bar is secured on the machine by two rotating hooks attached to the bar itself. After loading the bar and assuming the correct starting position, rotate the hooks forward to release the bar. Then lower the bar to the upper chest or trapezius area (depending on whether you choose to do military or behind-the-neck presses). The bar is limited to vertical movement only; the nature of the machine prevents any forward or backward movement.

DUMBBELL LATERAL RAISE

Muscles Used: Deltoid (primarily the lateral head), **supraspinatus**

Exercise Technique: Start with hands facing the legs, arms and dumbbells at the sides. Using only the shoulder musculature to lift, raise the weight until the arms are parallel to the floor. A slight bend at the elbow is permissible as long as the weight remains in line with the shoulder joint (Figure 10-4).

Fitness Tip

Spotting the Shoulder Press

When spotting the shoulder press the spotter should always be directly behind the lifter. In the case of the dumbbell shoulder press, the spotter's hands should be on the wrists of the lifter and should remain in contact through the set, lifting as necessary. With the barbell option the spotter should either spot under each elbow or on the bar itself (inside of the lifter's grip), lifting up when necessary. Always aid the lifter in taking the weight off (at the beginning) and replacing the weight (at the end) to minimize shoulder strain and lessen the chance of other mishaps.

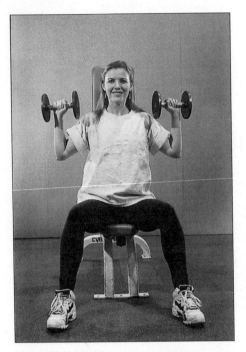
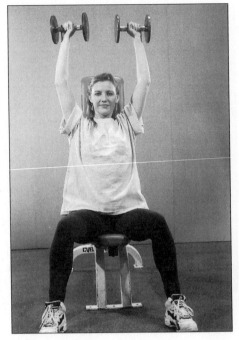

FIGURE 10-3 Shoulder press.

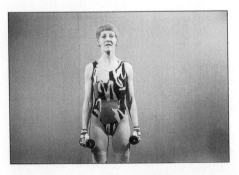
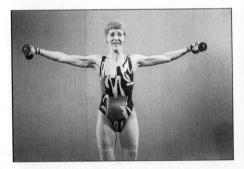

FIGURE 10-4 Dumbbell lateral raise.

DUMBBELL FRONT RAISE

Muscles Used: Deltoid (primarily the anterior head)

Exercise Technique: Hold the dumbbells in front of the body, with arms to the side and palms facing the torso. Without the aid of other muscles (such as leg swing), lift the weight until the arm is parallel to the floor and perpendicular to the torso. A barbell may be used for variation (Figure 10-5).

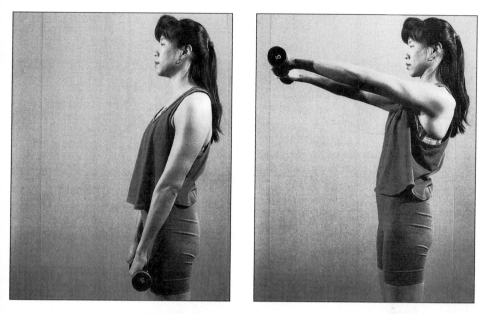

FIGURE 10-5 Dumbbell front raise.

ROTATOR CUFF EXERCISES

LYING EXTERNAL ROTATOR LIFT

Muscles Used: **Infraspinatus, teres minor**
Exercise Technique: Lie on your left side on a bench with the right arm at a 90 degree angle. Grasp the dumbbell with the right hand, palm facing the torso. A pad or the other hand may be placed under the elbow for stabilization. Begin with the arm below the waist and even with the right leg. From this position, elevate the arm while keeping the elbow stationary until the forearm is perpendicular to the torso. Always perform this and all single-limb exercises for both the left and right sides of the body (Figure 10-6).

SEATED INTERNAL ROTATOR LIFT

Muscles Used: **Subscapularis**
Exercise Technique: This exercise requires that the lifter sit on the floor or a bench holding a dumbbell on the side to be exercised. Grasp the dumbbell with the palm facing the opposite side of the body. The elbow is stationary and the forearm is extended away from the body. When exercising the left arm, pull the dumbbell across the body toward the right leg; perform the opposite motion when exercising the right arm (Figure 10-7).

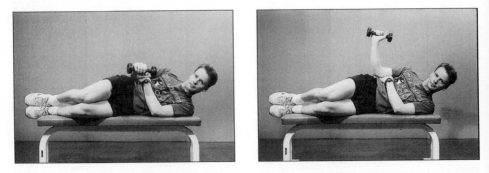

FIGURE 10-6 Lying external rotator lift.

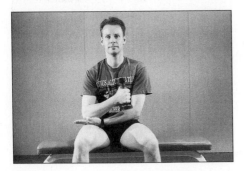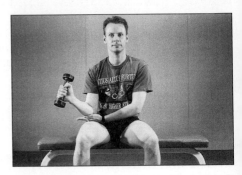

FIGURE 10-7 Seated internal rotator lift.

Fitness Tip

S.I.T.S.: The Rotator Cuff

The rotator cuff consists of four muscles: the subscapularis (internal rotator), the infraspinatus and teres minor (external rotator), and the supraspinatus (arm abductor worked in medial deltoid exercises). Hence the acronym S.I.T.S. These little muscles are critical in many activities. Among the activities most often associated with this area are baseball and softball, javelin, and tennis.

SUMMARY

- The trapezius raises, retracts, and rotates the scapula.
- The deltoid is the prime mover of arm abduction. It is also responsible for flexion and medial rotation of the humerus, and extension and lateral rotation of the arm.
- The four rotator cuff muscles are: supraspinatus, infraspinatus, teres minor, and subscapularis. An acronym to remember them by is S.I.T.S.
- Exercises for working the upper back and shoulder area include the following: upright row, shrug, shoulder press (dumbbell or barbell), Smith machine shoulder press, dumbbell lateral raise, dumbbell front raise, lying external rotator lift, and seated internal rotator lift.

▶ **Deltoid   p. 99**
Action: prime mover of arm abduction, flexion and medial rotation of upper arm (anterior head), extension and lateral rotation of arm (posterior head).

▶ **Infraspinatus   p. 103**
Action: rotates humerus laterally.

▶ **Subscapularis   p. 103**
Action: primary medial rotator of the humerus.

▶ **Supraspinatus   p. 101**
Action: stabilizes shoulder joint, helps to prevent downward dislocation of the humerus (upper arm bone).

▶ **Teres minor   p. 103**
Action: rotates humerus laterally.

▶ **Trapezius   p. 99**
Action: stabilizes, raises, retracts, and rotates the scapula.

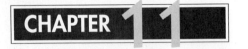

CHAPTER 11

LOWER BACK AND ABDOMINAL EXERCISES

OBJECTIVES

After reading this chapter, you should be able to do the following:

- Identify the major muscles of the middle and lower back and cite their primary functions.
- Identify the major abdominal muscles and cite their primary functions.
- Know several exercises for each of the previously identified muscles.

KEY TERMS

While reading this chapter, you will become familiar with the following terms:

► Erector Spinae Group
► External Oblique
► Internal Oblique

► Latissimus Dorsi
► Rectus Abdominis

More than 80 percent of all Americans will suffer from some sort of low back ailment in their lifetime. You can greatly decrease your chances of becoming part of this horrific statistic by taking several precautionary measures. First, engage in a regular flexibility program. Second, use correct biomechanical principles when lifting a load. Third, decrease excess body fat if your abdominal area is out of shape. This can be accomplished through a combination of dietary measures and aerobic exercise. Finally, strengthen your low back and abdominal musculature to aid in preventing injuries. This final point is what we will address in this chapter.

LOWER BACK EXERCISES

PULL-UP

Muscles Used: **Latissimus dorsi,** middle and lower trapezius

Exercise Technique: Take a shoulder width or slightly wider grip on the horizontal bar with the palms facing away from the body. The arms should be completely extended at this point, with the body hanging in a relaxed manner. From the extended position, pull the body up until the chin clears the bar. A wider grip restricts the range of motion and increases the difficulty of the exercise. A variation in which the lifter pulls up until the bar touches the upper shoulder area and the head is forward of the bar (behind-the-neck pull-ups) is also more difficult (Figure 11-1).

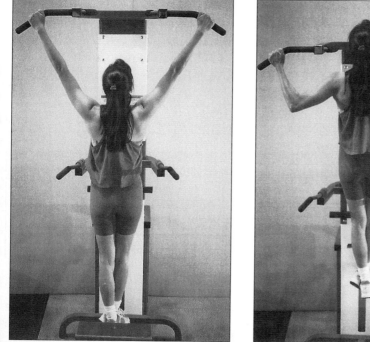
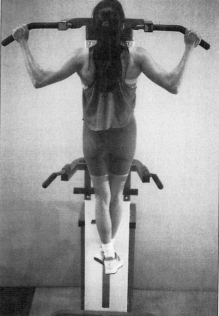

FIGURE 11-1 Pull-up.

Fitness Tip

Pull-Ups or Chin-Ups?

To perform chin-ups, the palms face the body and the biceps are involved, otherwise the movement is identical to pull-ups. As with dips, if you cannot perform the concentric (or pulling) motion, simply jump up and lower yourself slowly. Eventually this will give you more strength in the pulling phase of the movement.

LAT PULLDOWNS

Muscles Used: Latissimus dorsi, middle and lower trapezius

Exercise Technique: Sit at the lat pulldown station with the legs under and the knees slightly forward of the pads. The pads should be snug, but not tight on the legs. Extend the arms overhead to grasp the bar with a shoulder width grip, palms away from the body. Once again, this grip will work the muscles through a greater range of motion. The most common variation of this exercise is to bring the bar down until it touches the shoulders behind the neck. This variation can cause shoulder problems for some people. A less stressful variation is to bring the bar down to the front of the body to touch the upper chest area. While bringing the bar to the chest, lean back slightly, but still focus on keeping the back straight. Concentrate on driving the elbows down and back (Figure 11-2).

BENT-OVER ROWS

Muscles Used: Trapezius, latissimus dorsi, posterior deltoid, biceps brachii

Exercise Technique: To perform this exercise correctly it is imperative to keep the back almost parallel to the floor with the chest out and knees slightly bent. The torso should not sway back and forth on this movement. Bring the bar up from arm's length to touch the lower chest or rib cage area. When lowering the bar it is important to maintain tension in the muscles involved and not simply drop the bar.

BACK EXTENSION

Muscles Used: **Erector spinae group,** gluteus maximus

Exercise Technique: This exercise should be done on a specially designed bench, however, it may be done on any flat surface when raised a sufficient height from the

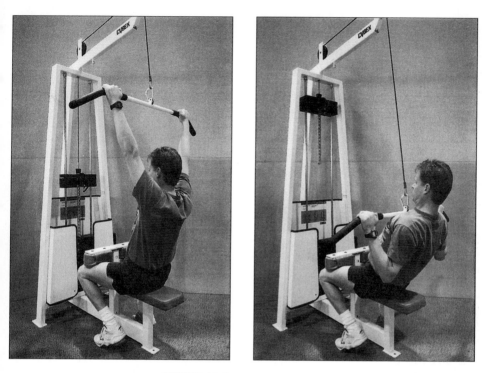

FIGURE 11-2 Lat pulldowns.

floor (a spotter will be needed to hold the feet). Lie facedown on the apparatus with the upper part of the hip area on the edge of the back extension bench. The arms may be crossed in front of the body or the fingers may be interlaced behind the head. The legs and hips remain motionless throughout the movement. Lower the upper body to a point between 45 and 90 degrees below the bench depending on your individual exercise tolerance (45 degrees is recommended for beginners). Then raise the body until it is parallel with the floor or is in 180 degree alignment. Do not exceed this point in the range of motion (Figure 11-3).

SEATED MACHINE ROW

Muscles Used: Trapezius, latissimus dorsi, posterior deltoid, biceps brachii

Exercise Technique: Seated at the rowing station, make certain that the seat is adjusted so that your shoulder joint and outstretched arms are in line with the machine handles. You may either grasp horizontally with elbows up and palms down, or vertically with thumbs up, hands neutral, and elbows down and in by your sides. Your chest should remain against the pad throughout the exercise. At this point, pull the handles back until your elbows just pass the back of your torso. Return to starting position.

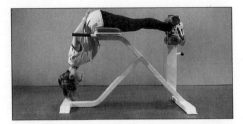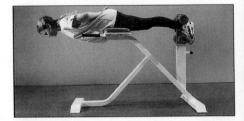

FIGURE 11-3 Back extension.

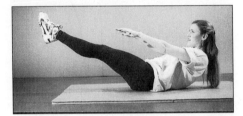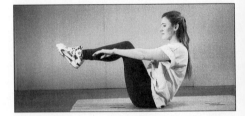

FIGURE 11-4 V-up.

ABDOMINAL EXERCISES

V-UP

Muscles Used: **Rectus abdominis,** iliopsoas

Exercise Technique: Begin by sitting on the floor with arms outstretched at each side. The legs should be extended (about 6 to 10 inches off the floor) with knees slightly bent. The arms are pulled back to a position by the pectoral muscles. Initiate movement by bringing the knees toward the torso and shooting the arms toward the ankles. Return to starting position and repeat as needed. Perform this movement slowly and with control (Figure 11-4).

CHINNIES

Muscles Used: Rectus abdominis, **internal oblique, external oblique**

Exercise Technique: Begin by lying on a pad (as with all abdominal floor work) with the legs extended and the hands interlocked behind the head. Flex the torso from the right side, extending the right elbow toward the left knee (which should come up simultaneously to meet the elbow). Return to starting position and repeat the procedure for the left side and right knee. This exercise takes a little time to develop, but once the rhythm is found it is a very useful movement (Figure 11-5).

HANGING KNEE RAISE

Muscles Used: Rectus abdominis, iliopsoas

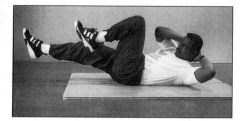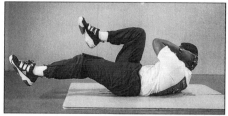

FIGURE 11-5 Chinnies.

Exercise Technique: Begin by holding yourself upright on your forearms on the knee raise station (keep a slight bend in the knees even in the extended position). From this point, bring the knees up until they are parallel with the floor. Slowly lower and repeat. It is critical that this exercise be done with control to prevent low back pain (Figure 11-6).

SUMMARY

- The latissimus dorsi is responsible for arm adduction and is the prime mover of arm extension.
- The erector spinae group extends the vertebral column and is responsible for maintaining erect posture.
- The internal and external obliques aid the muscles of the back in trunk rotation and lateral flexion.
- The rectus abdominis flexes and rotates the lumbar region of the vertebral column.
- Exercises for working the middle and lower back musculature include the following: pull-up, lat pulldown, bent-over row, back extension, and the seated machine row.
- Exercises for working the abdominal musculature include the following: v-up, chinnies, and hanging knee raise.

► **Erector Spinae Group   p. 108**
Action: extend vertebral column and maintain erect posture. Note that this group is comprised of three major back muscles: the iliocostalis, the longissimus, and the spinalis.

► **External Oblique   p.110**
Action: aids muscles of the back in trunk rotation and lateral flexion.

► **Internal Oblique   p. 110**
Action: aids muscles of the back in trunk rotation and lateral flexion.

► **Latissimus Dorsi   p. 107**
Action: arm adduction, prime mover of arm extension.

► **Rectus Abdominis   p. 110**
Action: flex and rotate lumbar region of vertebral column.

Fitness Tip

Maintaining Muscle Balance of the Lower Back and Abdominal Area

When training the lower back and abdominal area it is critical to remember their relationship. These two areas work synergistically in lifting loads and maintaining posture. It is of paramount importance that the beginning lifter realize this relationship and attempt to maintain a 1:1 strength ratio between the lower back and abdominal areas. This means that sets and reps should be approximated as closely as possible to be equal when working these two key muscle groups.

"The abdomen is the reason man does not easily take himself for a god."

—*Nietzsche*

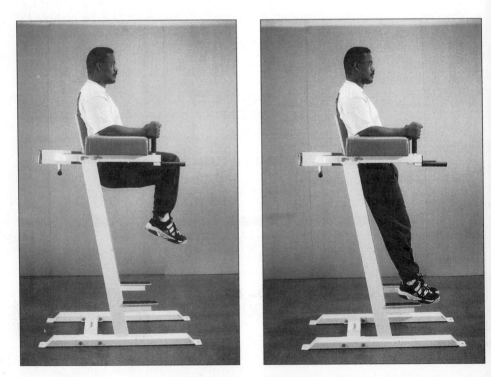

FIGURE 11-6 Hanging knee raise.

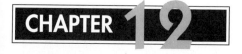

LEG EXERCISES

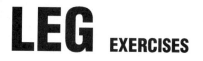

OBJECTIVES

After reading this chapter, you should be able to do the following:

- Identify the major muscles of the upper leg and cite their functions.
- Identify the major muscles of the lower leg and cite their functions.
- Know several exercises for each of the previously listed muscles.

KEY TERMS

While reading this chapter, you will become familiar with the following terms:

► **Adductor Brevis**

► **Adductor Magnus**

► **Gastrocnemius**

► **Gluteus Maximus**

► **Gluteus Medius**

► **Gluteus Minimus**

► **Gracilis**

► **Hamstring Group**

► **Iliopsoas**

► **Peroneus Longus**

► **Plantarflexion**

► **Quadricep Group**

Continued on p. 114.

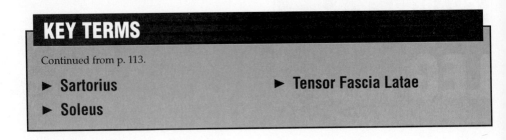

Continued from p. 113.

► **Sartorius**

► **Soleus**

► **Tensor Fascia Latae**

We have all heard the old cliches: "When your legs go, you go," "You're only as young as your legs," "Legs are the foundation on which the rest of your physique is built," etc. Texts as venerable as the Bible even make references to the importance of the legs: "when the guards of the house become shaky and the men of valor are bent . . ." (Ecclesiastes 12:3 JPS Version, 1985.) All of that being said, no one will deny the importance of firm and faithful underpinnings. Sports that rely on strong legs include: track and field, gymnastics, soccer, tennis, wrestling, competitive weight lifting, basketball, and football, to name a few. In everyday life, legs can often make or break us on the job. Whether we use them like the manual laborer or the floor nurse, the strength and endurance in our legs frequently determine how well we do our jobs and how we feel at the end of the day. Now that we have reinforced your image of the importance of your legs, let's start strengthening that shaky foundation!

LEG EXERCISES

SQUAT

Muscles Used: **Gluteus maximus,** quadriceps (the three vastii muscles in particular), hamstrings, gastrocnemius, erector spinae, **iliopsoas**

Exercise Technique: This exercise should not be done without a spotter, the use of a lifting belt, and sturdy squat stands or a power rack. Face the bar on the rack. Squat under it until the bar rests comfortably on the "traps," not the spinal cord in the neck region. Grasp the bar with a shoulder width or slightly wider grip. Standing erect, step back slowly and evenly from the stands until you are away from the pins. The feet should be shoulder width apart or slightly wider with the toes turned outward so that the knees track over the toes, reducing potential knee stress. Looking straight ahead squat down slowly and with control until the desired depth position is reached. Then reverse your drive and move back into the upright stance.

A good low position for beginners would be a 90 degree knee angle. Advanced squatters may go until the thighs are parallel with the floor. Ultimately depth will be determined by your ability to maintain correct form. Only go as low as you can handle with good form. Too much forward lean, rising up on your toes, and side to side motion during ascent or descent indicate that you should use a limited range of motion and less weight. Work on the form first, then increase the weight.

This is an exercise that should definitely be observed by a competent trainer for several sessions when first learning technique. The squat is one of the very best exercises for gaining size and strength, but it must be done correctly or it could be potentially harmful (Figure 12-1).

LUNGE

Muscles Used: Gluteus maximus, quadriceps, hamstrings, **adductor magnus, adductor brevis,** soleus

Exercise Technique: Assume the same starting hand and foot position that is used for the squat. With the barbell resting on the trapezius, step forward with either leg. Descend until a 90 degree angle is reached by the forward leg. The heel of the forward foot should be in line with the knee of the same leg to prevent excessive shear forces being generated on the knee. When descending use caution to avoid excessive forward lean of the torso. At the point of completing all of your prescribed repetitions for one leg, step back and repeat with the opposite leg.

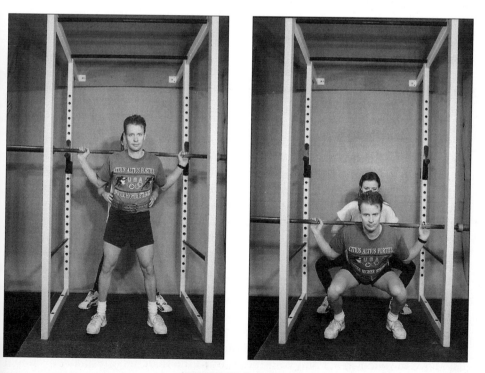

FIGURE 12-1 Squat.

Fitness Tip

Spotting the Squat

When only one spotter is available—one person should be sufficient unless you are attempting a maximum lift—the spotter should be positioned directly behind the lifter. Be prepared to lift up on the midtorso area if needed. Never grab the bar, as this could lead to loss of balance for the lifter. When going for a maximum limit lift, always use three spotters. Two should be on the outside, one on each end of the bar, and one should stand behind the lifter. It is very important that these three spotters work in sync when spotting, otherwise serious injuries could occur. If possible, squats should always be done inside a specially designed power rack. If spotters are not available and you must lift alone (not recommended), setting the pins at the correct height can save you if you fail in a squat attempt.

This exercise may also be performed while holding a dumbbell in each hand. Note: step-ups onto a sturdy bench with dumbbells in each hand are a possible substitute for this exercise, as the muscles involved are identical (Figure 12-2).

LEG OR KNEE EXTENSION

Muscles Used: **Quadricep group** (rectus femoris, vastus medialis, vastus intermedius, vastus lateralis)

Exercise Technique: Begin by sitting upright on the leg extension station. The knees should be in alignment with the machine's axis of rotation (the joint around which the movement arm rotates). The pads should make contact on your lower shin area. Bend the legs at a 90 degree angle and grasp the handles. From this position, extend the lower leg until it reaches a point almost parallel to the floor, but stopping short of hyperextension. Do not jerk or throw the weight (Figure 12-3).

LEG CURL OR KNEE FLEXION

Muscles Used: **Hamstring group** (semitendinosus, semimembranosus, biceps femoris), **sartorius**, gracilis

Exercise Technique: Begin lying facedown on the bench with knees in alignment with the axis of rotation and contacting the roller pad on the back of the lower leg just above the shoe area. Point your toes toward the floor and grasp any available handles. At this point, pull up the lower leg until it reaches a 90 degree angle at the

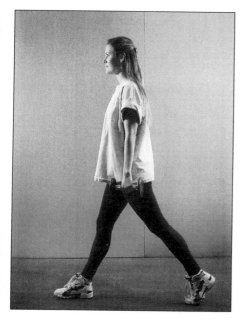
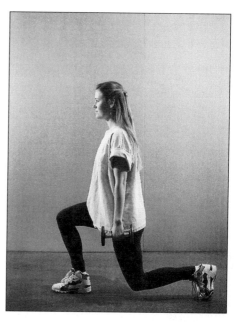

FIGURE 12-2 Lunge.

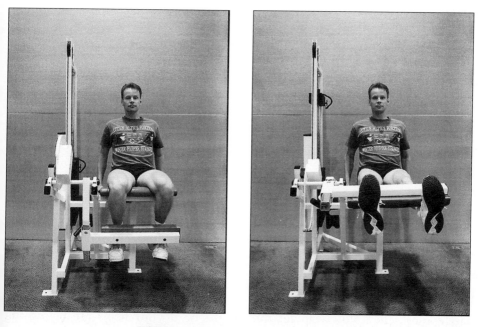

FIGURE 12-3 Leg or knee extension.

Fitness Tip

Maintaining Muscle Balance Between the Quadriceps and Hamstrings

The quadriceps and hamstrings are two groups where balance is crucial. Experts vary on the percentages, but most authorities state that the hamstring group should be 60 to 75 percent as strong (the actual weight lifted on a leg extension versus a leg curl) as the quadricep group. For some sports (i.e., cross-country skiing and sprinting in track and field) this ratio may approach a 1:1 relationship. One fact is certainly agreed upon: if a marked imbalance exists between the two groups, performance will suffer and the risk of injury rises.

knee. Then slowly lower the weight to its original position. Some benches are angled to aid in preventing back arching or lifting of the hips during this exercise. Both the leg curl and the leg extension may be performed with one leg at a time for rehabilitation or isolation purposes (Figure 12-4).

SEATED CALF RAISE

Muscles Used: **Soleus, peroneus longus**

Exercise Technique: This exercise can be performed with a machine or, lacking a machine, with a barbell wrapped in a towel placed over the lower quadricep area. If the machine is available, position yourself so that the pads contact the lower thighs just behind the knee. The ball of the foot should be placed on the platform with the heels lowered beneath the platform. From this position, rise up onto the balls of the feet to maximum height and then lower to the starting point. Do not go to the point of failure when doing this exercise, as it will be difficult to replace the safety bar under the movement arm (Figure 12-5).

STANDING CALF RAISE

Muscles Used: Medial and lateral **gastrocnemius,** soleus, peroneus longus

Exercise Technique: Position yourself under the pads so that they contact your shoulder area. At this point you should be standing upright and the weight stack on the calf raise machine should be directly in front of you. Rise up onto the balls of your feet until you can go no higher (**plantarflexion**). Then slowly lower the weight until your heels are below the platform height. On all calf exercises the goal should be high repetitions (on

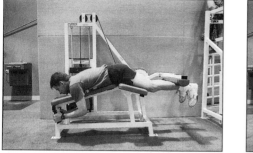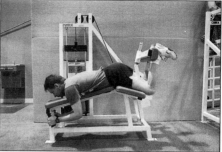

FIGURE 12-4 Leg curl or knee flexion.

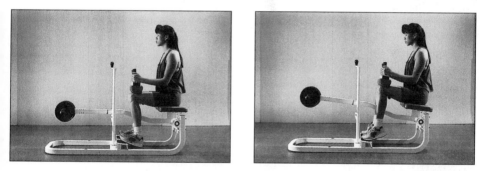

FIGURE 12-5 Seated calf raise.

the order of fifteen to twenty-five) with maximum weight. The combination of high reps and high weight will insure growth in this stubborn muscle group (Figure 12-6).

LEG PRESS

Muscles Used: Quadriceps (with the exception of the rectus femoris), hamstrings, gluteus maximus, adductor magnus, adductor brevis

Exercise Technique: Begin by sitting in the leg press station with the back pressed firmly against the torso pad and the feet on the moving platform. The feet should be shoulder width apart, with the toes turned slightly out, and the legs completely extended. Press up slightly to give the platform enough clearance to release the safety brakes. At this point, lower the weight with control until the knees reach a 90 degree angle and then press upward again until the starting position is regained. Avoid accelerating the platform to the point where it leaves the feet at the top of the range of motion (Figure 12-7).

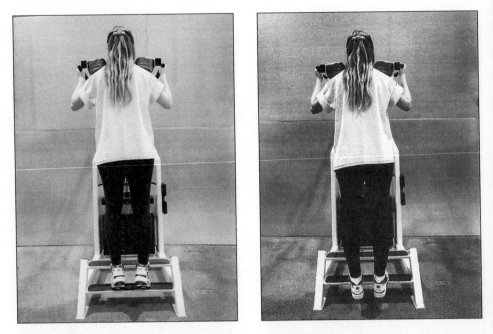

FIGURE 12-6 Standing calf raise.

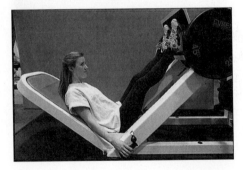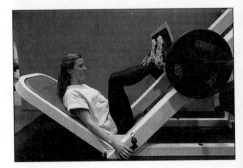

FIGURE 12-7 Leg press.

HIP ABDUCTION

Muscles Used: **Gluteus medius, gluteus minimus, tensor fascia latae**

Exercise Technique: For this exercise a multi-hip station will be needed (a low cable station with an attached leg strap may also be used). Position the pad on the outside of the leg just above the knee on the leg being exercised. The opposite leg supports the body in a standing position, torso upright, with the hip joint in alignment with the axis of rotation. The movement starts with the exercising leg in front of the supporting leg and to the left (for the right leg) by

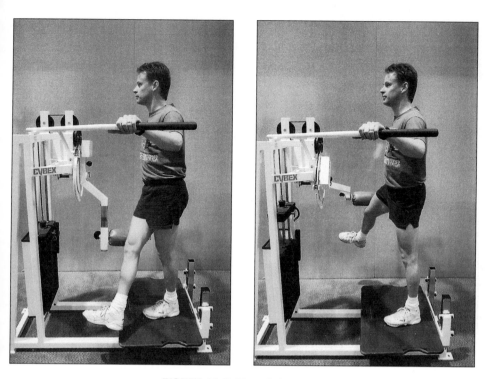

FIGURE 12-8 Hip abduction.

approximately 10 to 20 degrees. At this point, drive the leg, keeping the leg straight, out and away from the body until the limit of the range of motion is reached. Keep the torso upright throughout the movement. Be certain to exercise both legs equally (Figure 12-8).

HIP ADDUCTION

Muscles Used: Adductor magnus, **gracilis**

Exercise Technique: As for the previous exercise, this exercise also requires a multi-hip machine. Position the pad on the inside of the leg just above the knee on the leg being exercised. The opposite leg supports the body in a standing position, torso upright, with the hip joint in alignment with the axis of rotation. The movement starts with the exercising leg in front of the supporting leg and to the right (with the right leg being exercised). The right leg is extended to the limit of its abduction range of motion. From this point, the leg is pulled in until it crosses in front of the supporting leg (left leg) by approximately 10 to 20 degrees. Keep the torso upright throughout the movement. Be certain to exercise both legs equally (Figure 12-9).

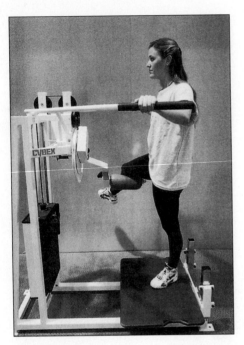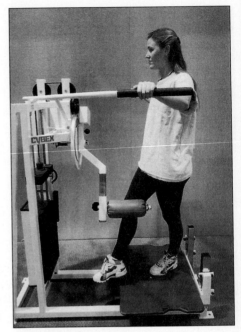

FIGURE 12-9 Hip adduction.

SUMMARY

- The gluteus maximus is the strongest muscle in the body and is a primary hip extensor.
- The quadriceps group acts as a knee extensor and hip flexor.
- The hamstring group acts as a knee flexor and hip extensor.
- The adductor magnus and adductor brevis are leg adductors.
- The gluteus minimus, gluteus medius, and tensor fascia latae are leg abductors.
- The iliopsoas (iliacus and psoas major) is the prime mover of hip flexion.
- The soleus, gastrocnemius, and peroneus longus are ankle plantar flexors.
- The sartorius flexes and laterally rotates the thigh.
- The gracilis adducts, flexes, and medially rotates the thigh.
- The knee extension works the frontal thigh musculature.
- The leg curl works the posterior thigh.
- Exercises for working the lower leg musculature include the seated calf raise and standing calf raise.
- Exercises for working the inner and outer thigh musculature include the hip abduction and hip adduction.
- Exercises for working all the major leg muscles include the squat, lunge, and leg press.

▶ **Adductor Brevis**   p. 115
Action: adducts and laterally rotates the thigh.

▶ **Adductor Magnus**   p. 115
Action: adducts and laterally rotates the thigh.

▶ **Gastrocnemius**   p. 118
Action: ankle plantar flexor when knee is extended.

▶ **Gluteus Maximus**   p. 114
Action: major hip extensor.

▶ **Gluteus Medius**   p. 120
Action: abducts and medially rotates the thigh.

▶ **Gluteus Minimus**   p. 120
Action: abducts and medially rotates the thigh.

▶ **Gracilis**   p. 121
Action: adducts thigh, flexes and medially rotates the leg.

▶ **Hamstring Group**   p. 116
Action: hip extension and knee flexion.

▶ **Iliopsoas**   p. 114
Action: hip flexor.

▶ **Peroneus Longus**   p. 118
Action: ankle plantar flexor, everts foot.

▶ **Plantarflexion**   p. 118
Pointing the toes downward, rising up on the toes.

▶ **Quadricep Group**   p. 116
Action: knee extension (all four muscles), hip flexion (rectus femoris).

▶ **Sartorius**   p. 116
Action: flexes and laterally rotates the thigh.

▶ **Soleus**   p. 118
Action: ankle plantar flexor (isolated only with bent knee).

▶ **Tensor Fascia Latae**   p. 120
Action: flexes and abducts thigh, rotates thigh medially.

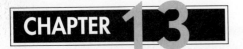

CHAPTER 13

SPECIAL EXERCISES AND ADVANCED CONCEPTS FOR HEALTH AND SPORT

> "It is those who dare danger and endure toil who achieve glorious deeds."
>
> —*Alexander the Great*

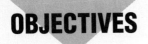

OBJECTIVES

After reading this chapter, you should be able to do the following:

- Identify the two Olympic lifts and be familiar with the basics of technique involved in the two lifts. Understand the usefulness of these lifts in various training programs.
- Identify the three powerlifts and be familiar with the basics of technique involved in the three lifts. Understand the usefulness of these lifts in various training programs.
- Understand a basic definition of plyometrics: what they are, how they work, and some sporting activities that might benefit from these drills.
- Understand what periodization is and how it can help you achieve your goals in a strength and conditioning program.
- Be conversant with several basic weight training programs for several popular and common sporting activities.
- Understand strength assessment: what it is, how it is performed, and how it can help you optimize progress in your workouts.

124

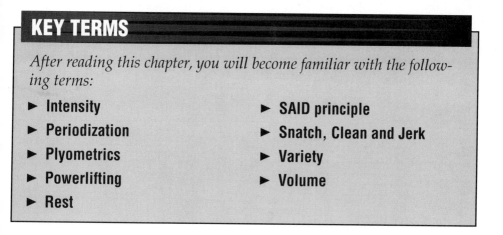

After reading this chapter, you will become familiar with the following terms:

► Intensity
► Periodization
► Plyometrics
► Powerlifting
► Rest

► SAID principle
► Snatch, Clean and Jerk
► Variety
► Volume

The concepts covered in this chapter go beyond the needs of most beginning trainees. That being said, there are concepts in this chapter that can be of benefit to everyone. However, most of the topics that we will touch on here relate to skills and methods that would aid the intermediate or advanced lifter. Novice strength coaches could also expand their working knowledge of techniques with the advice in this section. Most of what you will find in this chapter has been distilled from years of field research and trial and error methods that have yielded proven avenues to improving strength, power, and overall fitness. If you have passed the beginner stage and are looking for ways to keep improving or entertaining thoughts of competitive lifting, read on.

THE OLYMPIC LIFTS

The **snatch** and the **clean and jerk** are the only two Olympic lifts presently contested (the press was dropped from the program due to excessive arching on the lift). Both of these lifts are dynamic, explosive movements that involve all of the major muscles of the body in a fluid expression of power output. The highest power outputs ever measured in humans have been recorded during the performance of Olympic lifts. The lifts are, however, very complex and take years to master completely. They should not be attempted without the supervision of a qualified (USWF or NSCA certified) coach who can help identify technique flaws and decrease the likelihood of injury. For more information on learning these lifts and finding qualified coaches contact the USWF (United States Weightlifting Federation) or the NSCA (National Strength and Conditioning Association), both of which are located in Colorado Springs, Colorado.

When learning both the snatch and the clean and jerk it is best to start with the snatch. Learn the technique with a broomstick first and then progress to a barbell. Start by learning the hang snatch (from above the knees) and then progress to the complete movement. Learning to pull from the knees first will help avoid having to learn the "scoop," or second pull, after learning the pull from the floor. The "scoop" or second pull is a much more difficult progression to master. Try learning the Olympic lifts in the following manner.

SNATCH

1. Shrug with the bar. As the arms remain straight, shrug shoulders to the ears.
2. High pull from the hang position. Pull the bar to a high chest position.
3. Complete the pull from the hang to an overhead lockout.
4. Learn the starting position for the snatch pull from the floor.
5. Learn the pull from the floor and the complete snatch movement (Figure 13-1).

CLEAN AND JERK

1. Learn the rack position.
2. Work on the dip for the jerk.
3. Jerk from the rack position.

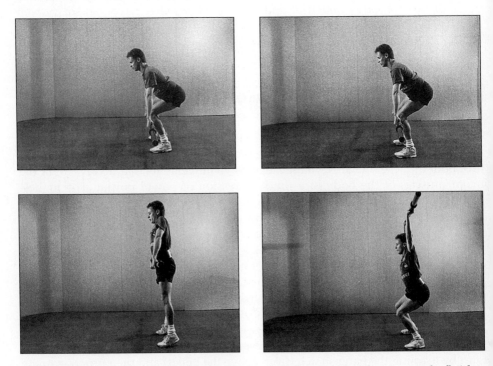

FIGURE 13-1 Proper form in learning the snatch is needed for a smooth, fluid motion throughout.

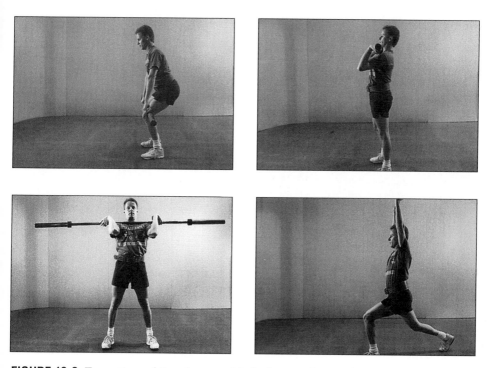

FIGURE 13-2 Execution of the clean and jerk. Instruction and coaching are needed to ensure proper technique.

4. Pull from the hang to the clean rack.
5. Learn the starting position for the clean pull from the floor.
6. Learn the clean pull from the floor and the complete clean and jerk movement (Figure 13-2).

THE POWERLIFTS

Powerlifting consists of three lifts, contested in this order: the squat, the bench press, and the deadlift. Each contestant is allowed three attempts for each of the three lifts, or nine lifts total. The idea is to start with a weight high enough so that you improve, but not so high that you fail to make your openers. As in Olympic lifting, once you have chosen your opener you may not go lower in weight. For example if you fail to get your opening squat you may either repeat it on your second attempt or go to a higher weight. The mechanics of the squat and bench press have been covered earlier in this book. For specifics on the deadlift, see the following box.

PLYOMETRICS

Plyometrics in some form or another has existed since the dawn of time. The ancient Greek pentathlon included jumping as an integral part of its five-event

The Deadlift

Muscles Used: Gluteus maximus, hamstrings, erector spinae, latissimus dorsi

Exercise Technique: The deadlift is a very complete and demanding exercise. Do not attempt to learn this exercise until you have several years of training under your belt and you have an expert coach to give you feedback on technique. Do not do this exercise if you have a history of back problems. The deadlift is not for everyone, but if you find that you can do it, the iron bug will probably bite hard and you are likely to stay with this challenging exercise. More weight has been lifted in this exercise than in any other squat. There is a fundamental joy in being able to pull a heavy weight off the ground!

Start by learning this exercise with a light weight and determining which stance [close (arms outside the legs) or sumo (legs outside the arms)] will work best for you. Whole books have been written on powerlifting techniques, so if this little vignette intrigues you, research it further.

In learning the basics it is imperative that you start with the bar over the balls of your feet, or closer, hands about thumb's width from the inside knurling, and reversed. One hand (usually the dominant) has the palm facing the torso and the other has the palm facing away. For the sake of simplicity, the sumo technique will be described here as it is the one this author is most familiar with in competition. The head is in the neutral position and the back is straight, yet slightly convex. The shoulders should be up and over the front of the bar.

From this position, the lifter drives the legs down into the floor and pulls the shoulders up. The arms never bend and the lifter should fight the tendency to lift the glutes or buttocks prematurely as this will put the back in a vulnerable position. Continue to drive the legs and pull the bar up until the upright position is reached with the bar at the mid- or upper thigh position.

To replace the bar on the floor it is necessary to reverse the aforementioned procedure with great care and control of body alignment. Remember, a coach should give you feedback on your form while performing this lift.

If you are interested in powerlifting, seek out your local governing body (USPF, IPF, ADFPA) or simply ask your county recreation office if they conduct any powerlifting meets. Do not be afraid to get involved because you don't think that you are strong enough. Everyone has to start with that first awkward meet. Be certain to get a physical from your physician before entering any competitive lifting meets (Figure 13-3).

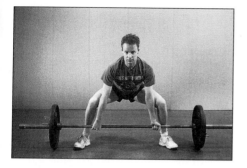 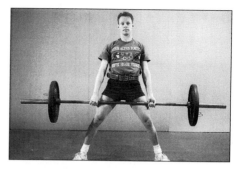

FIGURE 13-3 The deadlift should not be attempted until you have several years of training under your belt.

program. The educational classic *Gargantua and Pantagruel* by Rabelais includes the use of many jumping and throwing drills in the physical preparation of the young giant. In the Renaissance period Mercurialis included a chapter on the medical effects of jumping in his work *The Art of Gymnastics.* Also in this time period Tuccaro, a court acrobat and gymnast, wrote *Three Dialogues on the Art of Jumping.* The first modern manual of physical education, *Gymnastics for Youth,* written by GutsMuths in 1793, included a chapter on jumping exercises. The twentieth-century conception of plyometrics as we have come to know it today was developed in the former Soviet Union by track coaches and researchers. Verhoshanski performed much of the early research on bounding and depth jumps. The American track and field writer Fred Wilt first introduced the term and its basic concepts to the Western world in 1976. Since then other pioneers like Gambetta and Chu have written numerous articles on this subject. Two basic definitions of plyometrics include the following:

> "Elastic strength is that type of strength where both the contractile and elastic components are assisted by the stretch reflex contraction in the expression of strength at speed."
>
> *Dick, 1984*

> "This means that during eccentric or negative work, elastic energy is stored within the muscles to be reused during the following concentric or positive phase in the form of mechanical work which in turn improves performance."
>
> *Bosco, 1982*

Simply stated, plyometric drills help to bridge the gap between strength training and pure power. In the author's masters thesis (Field, 1987), a twice weekly commitment of ten minutes to plyometric drills produced an average improvement of 3 inches in the vertical jump of male volleyball and basketball players and an average of 2 inches in female athletes.

BASIC PLYOMETRICS TERMINOLOGY

1. Jump: consists of a two-foot landing
2. Hop: consists of a one-foot landing on the same leg

Fitness Tip

Before You Start Plyometrics

1. Proper footwear. Wear sturdy, flexible shoes.
2. Resilient surface. Exercise on grass, sawdust, a gymnastic floor, or wrestling mats. No concrete or basketball courts!
3. Equipment. Assemble anything you might need for drills (i.e., boxes, medicine balls, cones).
4. Preparation. Begin with a general thorough specific warm up.
5. Technique considerations. Stop any exercise as soon as technique starts to break down!
6. Progression. Follow the progressions outlined in section II of the following outline.
7. Training/biological age. Do not attempt to do exercises that are beyond your physical age limits (i.e., a twelve-year-old athlete should not be doing depth jumps or high volume hopping). The training age is the number of years that an athlete has been training for a specific activity. An athlete with a higher training age can attempt more difficult drills if other factors do not contraindicate the use of such exercises.
8. Weight. Athletes using weights over 200 lbs. should use extreme caution with moderate to high level drills. Greater weight will cause greater stress on joints, tendons, and muscle tissue.
9. Injuries. The athlete's prior injury history should be carefully considered prior to the selection and use of plyometric exercises.
10. Fatigue. Athletes should be continually monitored for fatigue. Plyometric exercises should not be performed when the athlete is fatigued or highly stressed. These exercises will yield the greatest benefits when the athlete is rested and fresh.

3. Bound: consists of moving from one foot to another
4. In-place jump: activity that is performed in the same location
5. Short jump: activity with 10 repetitions or less
6. Long jump: activity with 10 or more repetitions
7. Shock method: activity with a high central nervous system stress, which greatly taxes the athlete

GETTING STARTED WITH PLYOMETRICS

I. When using the NSCA plyometric continuum
   A. Low level drills are appropriate for beginners.
   B. Low to medium level drills are appropriate for the intermediate level athlete.
   C. Medium to shock level drills are appropriate for the advanced or elite level athlete.

II. Progression
   A. Low intensity to high intensity
   B. Slow-moving drills to fast-moving drills
   C. In-place drills to drills with movement
   D. Double- to single-leg or multiple movements
   E. Shock method drills (very high intensity and complexity)
   F. General to athletically specific tasks

III. NSCA beginner physical prerequisite recommendations
   A. 5 push-ups
   B. 5 squat thrusts
   C. Standing long jump equal to one's height
   D. Jump rope for 30 seconds
   E. Square pattern jumping and hopping

IV. **Volume** considerations
   A. Contacts: number of times a body part meets the ground (i.e., footstrikes)
      1. Beginner: 50–100 contacts daily/two times per week
      2. Intermediate: 100–200 contacts daily/two times per week
      3. Elite: 150–300 contacts daily/two to three times per week
   B. Distance covered

V. Volume versus **intensity** relationship
   A. There is an inverse relationship between these two variables and they must be closely balanced to prevent overtraining and optimize performance.
   B. Intensity in plyometrics may be gauged by the progression (see section II). For example, drill IIa is lower in intensity than drill IId. In weight lifting, intensity is directly related to the weight on the bar. The higher the weight, the higher the intensity. The number of reps at a given weight can also factor into the computation of intensity.

VI. When to use plyometric drills in a workout
   A. After a thorough general and specific warm up
   B. Generally before weight training, although plyometrics can be interspersed throughout a weight session by a knowledgeable trainer
   C. Before running training
   D. Before or after technique work as long as the technique work is not of a highly fatiguing nature

VII. Plyometric testing drills*
   A. Total body
      1. Overhead backward shot throw
      2. Underhand forward shot throw
   B. Lower body
      1. Standing long jump
      2. Standing three continuous long jumps
      3. Five single-leg bounds with an approach
   C. Upper body
      1. Medicine ball put while seated, one- and two-arm
      2. Clap push-ups

*Note: For norms on these and other plyometric drills please consult the jumps decathlon table (V. Gambetta, Ed. *TAC Coaching Manual*, 1989, Leisure Press) and *NSCA Journal* articles such as Volume 13, No. 3, 1991, p. 50.

PERIODIZATION

A simple definition of **periodization** would be the planning of varied training principles so that the lifter is able to exceed previous best performances. The term *periodization* comes from the the use of "periods" or phases of the training cycle. Traditionally, the annual training cycle has been divided into three main segments: preparatory or preseason, competitive or in-season, and transition or off-season. Depending on the sport involved, the number of peaks and their spacings throughout the year will vary.

This section could be termed "doing more with less," as it deals with the manipulation of training volumes and intensities to maximize performance. Too many coaches and athletes think that more is always better and grind themselves into a permanent state of overtraining. There are many hard trainers who would make much greater gains in size and strength if they used lesser training volumes and cycled intensity, and took more frequent and longer rest periods between workouts. The origins of this training theory can be traced to researchers Leo Matveyev and Tudor Bompa, hailing from Russia and Romania respectively. Their theories of adaptation to stressors were based on that of Hans Selye's general adaptation syndrome.

PERIODIZATION TERMINOLOGY

1. Macrocycle: usually a year in time although it can be a period of several years or several months
2. Mesocycle (also spelled "mezzocycle"): a period of several months or an extended length of time in weeks (i.e., 16 weeks)
3. Microcycle: one week
4. Units: a training session within a day; each day may contain more than one training unit
5. Supercompensation: the theory that by applying optimal stress to the body and giving sufficient recovery time, the body will come back at a higher functional state
6. **SAID principle:** specific adaptation to imposed demands
7. Hypertrophy phase: the phase where size growth and high volume, low-intensity training is stressed (50 to 75 percent one-repetition maximum and 8–12 repetitions)
8. Strength phase: the phase where volume begins to moderate as intensity rises (80 to 90 percent one-repetition maximum and 5–8 repetitions)
9. Power phase (also known as the competition phase): phase at which intensity reaches its peak while volume is minimized (90 to 100+ percent and 1–4 repetitions). A one- or two-week maintenance phase may be inserted at this point.
10. Transition or active rest phase: in this phase, which can last anywhere from one week to one month, the athlete regenerates the body by not lifting and utilizing other activities as active recovery.

TABLE 13-1
Periodization Example 1: Strength/Power

Week	Reps	Sets	Weight (lbs.) (Leg Press)
1	5	5	100
2	4	4	110
3	3	3	120
4	5	5	110
5	4	4	120
6	3	4	130

TABLE 13-2
Periodization Example 2: The Hypertrophy Phase

Week	Reps	Sets	Weight (lbs.) (Chest Press)
1	12	4	100
2	10	3	105
3	8	3	110
4	6	3	100
5	12	4	105
6	10	3	110
7	8	3	115
8	6	3	105

So how does periodization work? This topic can become quite complex and texts have been written on this subject, several excellent ones by Tudor Bompa. To keep it simple, here are two working examples of periodization in a strength training cycle. This first cycle is a crossover from the strength/power phase (Table 13-1). Looking at this simple, yet truly effective cycle will show that: (1) the weight increased as the reps decreased, and (2) the weight increased when going through the cycle for the second time.

On week 1 the target weight is 100 lbs. for five sets of five reps. The next time five sets of five reps are performed is in week 4, and the weight is now 110 lbs. Keep in mind that individuals will vary in how much they can increase in weight. The aforementioned chart is intended to be used as a guide.

The second cycle example is from the hypertrophy phase and would be appropriate for bodybuilding applications as well as strength training (Table 13-2).

Again in this example the weight increases with a drop in repetitions, and the second cycle increases the weight for the same reps and sets. However, this cycle utilizes two "unloading" weeks (weeks 2 and 8) in which both the volume and intensity are low prior to going back into the cycle again. This allows the body to supercompensate and to renew itself in order to lessen the chance of overtraining.

This is a good point to insert several critical words of advice. Do not attempt to mimic the routines of champions. Many of them have trained for years and have a greater training base and more experience. Some have the help of anabolic steroids and other ergogenic aids. Attempting to follow their programs will lead to overtraining, failure, and perhaps quitting altogether. Excellent gains can be made on abbreviated programs (e.g., two to five exercises per workout, two to three times per week). Some top lifters train each muscle group only once a week. Some top powerlifters now train squat and bench once a week and deadlift once every two weeks, and they are among the best in the world! Realize that the intensity in these cases is very high and that several days recovery (not just forty-eight hours) is necessary.

Intensity is the key to strength training progress. All the volume in the world won't help you if your intensity is too low. Emphasize quality, not quantity. Keep in mind the inverse relationship between volume and intensity: if one is high, the other cannot be high without leading to overtraining or injuries. If you understand the relationships between volume and intensity, and work and recovery, you'll be light years ahead of your training partners.

Save the split routines and twice a day training for the genetically gifted and those with no other jobs or responsibilities! Try to keep your workout times under one hour each session and focus on major, multijoint exercises such as the squat, bench press, military press or press behind the neck, shrugs, and deadlift (if you can handle it). Many of the top strength and physique stars in the world have made excellent gains on these abbreviated programs and they will work much better for the average trainee. The newest routine of Mr. or Ms. Galaxy will destroy the hopes and recovery ability of 95 percent of the weight trainers in "real world" (drug free, jobs, school, etc.) conditions. In other words, the published routines of most national and international bodybuilders and weight trainers are inappropriate for the average trainee. Keep in mind that if you are training hard and not seeing strength or size gains, you may need to train less, not more. In the words of Mike Mentzer (1978 Mr. Universe who trained with abbreviated programs) the keys to training success are keeping exercise (1) intense, (2) brief, and (3) infrequent (*Heavy Duty*, Mentzer, 1993). However, do not interpret this to mean one should train only once a week or once every two weeks.

REST AND VARIETY

Rest and variety are two keys to long-term progress and exercise adherence. **Rest** can be as simple as the time you take between sets (30 seconds for muscular endurance, 30–90 seconds for mass building, or 3–5 minutes for strength gains) or as complex as the rest periods between workouts that we've just discussed. The key is to find out what works for you. Listen to your body. If you are still hurting from yesterday's workout, you have not recovered!

Variety is another big key to long-term progress and just sticking with a program. Change your routines every six to eight weeks. Change the order, change the days you work out on, change the actual exercises, change your workout time, change the place where you work out. Are you getting the picture yet? The number one reason trainees drop out is boredom. With all the options available to today's lifters this should not be happening. If your training works and you are progressing, stick with it. If you have stalled out, change your routine now! Evaluate your program logically, based on your goals, time constraints, training state, social commitments, and budgetary restrictions. Remember to listen to your body. It is your own best coach!

> "If you desire a powerful body then you must train it with gymnastics in sweat and labor"
>
> —*Virtue to Heracles*

▶ **Intensity   p. 131**
A measure of the CNS (central nervous system) fatigue and therefore systemic or total body fatigue.

▶ **Periodization   p. 132**
The planning of varied training principles so that the lifter is able to exceed previous best performances. The term periodization comes from the the use of "periods" or phases of the training cycle. Traditionally the annual training cycle has been divided into three main segments: preparatory or pre-season, competitive or in-season, and transition or off-season.

▶ **Plyometrics   p. 127**
An exercise technique that uses elastic strength where both the contractile and elastic components of the muscle are assisted by the stretch reflex contraction in the expression of strength at speed.

▶ **Powerlifting   p. 127**
Three lifts, contested in this order: the squat, the bench press, and the deadlift.

▶ **Rest   p. 134**
The time you take between sets or the rest periods between workouts.

▶ **SAID Principle   p. 132**
Specific adaptation to imposed demands.

▶ **Snatch and Clean and Jerk   p. 125**
The only two Olympic lifts presently contested (the press was dropped from the program due to excessive arching on the lift).

▶ **Variety   p. 135**
Changing the order, schedule, exercises, etc., of your workout routine to avoid boredom.

▶ **Volume   p. 131**
The amount of exercise in a program; measured in contacts or distance covered in plyometric work. Volume is measured by multiplying reps times sets in weight lifting to give a picture of the total workload.

PROGRAMS FOR SELECTED SPORTS

The following are sample programs for several popular sports. Two options are presented: free weight and machine. Choose one or the other or combine exercises from each column. Try, however, to avoid doing multiple exercises for the same muscle group area.

SOCCER

	Free weight	Machine (using Cybex terminology)
Off-season (2–3 sets of 8–12 reps)	Lunge	Leg press
	Standing leg curl	Lying leg curl
	One-leg calf raise	Standing calf raise
	Dumbbell row	Lat pulldown
	Dumbbell bench	Chest press
	Shrug	Shoulder press
	Dumbbell curl	Biceps curl
	Triceps extension	Triceps pushdown
	Crunch	Modular abdominal
	Back extension	Modular low back
In-season (1–2 sets of 4–6 reps)	Power clean	Leg press
	Step-ups	Lat pulldown
	Incline bench	Chest press
	Crunch	Modular abdominal

Note: Abs can be done separately as another part of the program.

BASKETBALL

	Free weight	Machine
Off-season (2–3 sets of 8–12 reps)	Squats	Incline leg press
	Lying leg curl	Seated leg curl
	Donkey calf raise	Standing calf raise
	Seated barbell calf raise	Seated calf raise
	Bent-over row	Seated row
	Flat bench	Pec-dec
	Upright row	Lateral raise
	EZ curl	Pulley curl
	Close-grip bench	Triceps extension
	Knee raise	Seated oblique

In-season (1–2 sets of 4–6 reps)	High pull	Super cat (special weight machine designed for improving vertical leap)
	Dumbbell squat	Seated row
	Dip	Machine fly
	Back extension	Modular low back

SWIMMING

Off-season (2–3 sets of 12–25 reps)	Free weight	Machine
	Dumbbell lunge	Hack squat
	One-leg lying leg curl	One-leg lying leg curl
	Standing calf raise	Calf press on the leg press machine
	Pull-up	T-bar row
	Dip	Pec-dec
	Dumbbell fly	Cable crossover
	Dumbbell rotator exercises	Cable rotator exercises
	Concentration curl	One-arm cable curl
	Seated one-arm overhead triceps extension	Overhead triceps extension with rope
	Reverse crunch	Russian twist on bench
In-season (1-2 sets of 6-10 reps)	Lunge	Incline leg press
	Pull-up	Close-grip pulldown
	Bench dip	Incline chest press
	Handstand push-up	Lateral raise
	Crunch	Rope ab crunches

SUMMARY

- The snatch and the clean and jerk are the two Olympic lifts presently contested. These lifts and their variations are very useful in producing power gains.
- The squat, bench press, and deadlift are the three lifts contested in powerlifting. These core lifts are very useful in the development of basic strength.
- Plyometrics is a form of training that improves explosive power. This method can involve upper and lower body exercises and is very dynamic in nature.
- Periodization or cycling involves the planning of performance cycles so that volume and intensity match the goals of a specific training phase.
- Weight training can be an effective adjunct to any athletic activity. Sample programs for some popular sports may be found in this chapter.

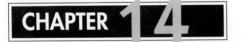

ANABOLIC **STEROIDS** AND OTHER **ERGOGENIC** AIDS

▼ OBJECTIVES

After reading this chapter, you should be able to do the following:

- List the five classifications of ergogenic aids.
- Understand why good nutrition is essential to strength development and athletic performance.
- List the side effects and health risks of taking anabolic steroids.

KEY TERMS

While reading this chapter, you will become familiar with the following terms:

► Amino Acid Supplements   ► Carbohydrate Loading

► Amphetamines   ► Ergogenic Aid

► Anabolic Steroids   ► Growth Hormone

Since the inception of structured weight training and bodybuilding people have been devising ways to gain more strength beyond that possible from weight training. Some people are willing to risk their health and their lives to get bigger, stronger, and perform better. Many athletes have been seriously injured and even killed as a result of taking illegal drugs to enhance their performance. The bottom line is it's just not worth the risk. You don't need to take drugs to get stronger or to be a successful athlete. Taking legal or illegal drugs to enhance your training will only hurt you in the long run.

ERGOGENIC AIDS

An **ergogenic aid,** simply defined, is any substance, process, or procedure that may, or is perceived to, enhance performance through improved strength, speed, response time, or endurance. Ergogenic aids can be broken down into five classifications: nutritional aids, physiological aids, psychological aids, pharmacological aids, and mechanical and biomechanical aids. Athletes have been using various forms of ergogenic aids for years, probably dating back to the first Olympics. It is common knowledge that the Incas chewed cocoa leaves in order to sustain strenuous work.

Some ergogenic aids are clearly safe and appropriate, such as, training methods, use of water, improved equipment, carbohydrate loading, warm-up techniques, mental relaxation techniques, and cool-down techniques. Other ergogenic aids are clearly illegal and against all the principles of the spirit of competition. Aids such as anabolic steroids, amphetamines, and other agents are illegal and pose a health risk to the athlete. Regardless of the lack of reliable research to prove the safety and effectiveness of certain ergogenic aids, athletes will continue to use them, and manufacturers will continue to develop new legal and illegal athletic aids.

DRUGS IN SPORTS

There is a variety of reasons why athletes take nonprescribed drugs. Some take drugs to feel better, to do better, or because others have told them to do so. The list goes on and on. However, there really is no good reason to risk your health, life, and career. No one wants to see an athlete's career ruined by illegal drug use. The only way to help prevent athletes from experimenting with or abusing drugs is to educate them. This chapter discusses some of the common drugs used by strength and weight training athletes.

ANABOLIC STEROIDS

Anabolic steroids are natural hormones formed in the testes and the adrenal glands. Steroid hormones make it easier for some cells to form additional protein. Steroids increase the rate at which muscle gains and tissue repair occur. A natural steroid, testosterone, produces two major effects on the body, androgenic and anabolic. Androgenic effects are responsible for the development of secondary sex characteristics (male facial hair and a deeper voice). Anabolic changes include the

Fitness Tip

Major Side Effects and Health Risks of Anabolic Steroids

Liver cancer	Breast enlargement (males)
Acne	Breast shrinkage (females)
Baldness	Deeper voice (females)
Increased body hair	Prostate cancer
Increased nervousness	Dizziness
Decreased testosterone production	Nosebleeds
Increased risk of heart disease	Increased aggressiveness
Leukemia	Increased urine production
Headaches	Water retention
Gastrointestinal problems	Oily skin
High blood pressure	Muscle cramps
Menstrual problems	Kidney damage
High cholesterol and triglycerides	

growth and development of certain body tissues, such as the rapid increase in muscle during puberty. Thus athletes search for the right mix of steroids to maximize the anabolic effects and minimize the androgenic effects. Nevertheless, all anabolic steroids produce some androgenic effects. The above Fitness Tip lists the major side effects and health risks of taking anabolic steroids.

Synthetic steroids were developed to treat certain forms of anemia and osteoporosis and for the prevention of muscle wasting in certain diseases. Synthetic steroids are routinely prescribed to promote tissue growth in patients who have had to remain in bed for an extended period of time. Synthetic steroids, which can only be prescribed by a physician, are now readily available on the black market, and have found their way into locker rooms and gyms. It has been reported that 90 percent of male athletes in sports such as weight lifting, power-lifting, and bodybuilding have used or will use steroids at some point in their career.

Do steroids work? The answer is yes. In conjunction with hard work or exercise, steroids have been shown to increase strength and muscle mass, but studies are inconsistent in their findings. Some studies have shown that equal amounts of strength and muscle mass gains can be achieved through high-intensity training and proper nutrition versus using steroids. So why do people keep taking some-

Fitness Tip

American College of Sports Medicine's Position on Anabolic Steroids

The American College of Sports Medicine, one of the most respected professional exercise and sports organizations, has published a position stand on anabolic-androgenic steroids based on a comprehensive literature review. According to the American College of Sports Medicine:

The administration of anabolic-androgenic steroids to healthy humans below age 50 in medically approved therapeutic doses often does not of itself bring about any significant improvements in strength, aerobic endurance, lean body mass, or body weight.

There is no conclusive scientific evidence that extremely large doses of anabolic-androgenic steroids either aid or hinder athletic performance.

The prolonged use of oral anabolic-androgenic steroids has resulted in liver disorders in some persons. Some of these disorders are apparently reversible with the cessation of drug usage, but others are not.

The administration of anabolic-androgenic steroids to male humans may result in a decrease in testicular size and function and a decrease in sperm production. Although these effects appear to be reversible when small doses of steroids are used for short periods of time, the reversibility of the effects of large doses over extended periods of time is unclear.

Serious and continuing efforts should be made to educate male and female athletes, coaches, physical educators, physicians, trainers, and the general public regarding the inconsistent effects of anabolic-androgenic steroids on improvement of human physical performance and the potential dangers of taking certain forms of these substances, especially in large doses, for prolonged periods of time.

(American College of Sports Medicine, 1994)

thing that involves more risks than benefits? Most people who take steroids are unaware of the risks involved. Steroids are illegal, and should not be taken without medical supervision. When you buy a drug off the street you have no idea what is in it, where it was manufactured, or how it has been processed and handled. Can you imagine injecting something into your body when you have no idea what is in it, or where or how it was produced?

The bottom line is, the potential benefits of taking steroids do not outweigh the potential risks. In addition, research has been inconsistent in demonstrating their effectiveness.

GROWTH HORMONE

Growth hormone is a protein secreted by the pituitary gland. Growth hormone helps support growth and the development of body tissues. It has only been within the last twenty years that a safe synthetic hormone has been available. Synthetic hormones are often given to children to stimulate growth. Although some athletes take growth hormone in an effort to stimulate muscle growth, little research is available to substantiate its use. Athletes often mix anabolic steroids with synthetic growth hormone to either enhance the overall effect of both drugs or to minimize the effect of one of the drugs. This procedure is referred to as "stacking."

AMPHETAMINES

Amphetamines are synthetic structured drugs similar to the naturally occurring chemical in our body called epinephrine. Like epinephrine, they produce stimulation of the central nervous system resulting in increased alertness in motor and physical activity, decrease in fatigue, and sometimes insomnia. Once again, research has found conflicting evidence regarding the effect of amphetamines on performance. To date, no studies have conclusively demonstrated that taking amphetamines improves strength or athletic performance. Amphetamines have been banned by the International Olympic Committee. As with steroids, the risks of taking amphetamines outweigh the potential benefits. The following Fitness Tip lists the health and side effects of amphetamine use.

Fitness Tip

Health and Side Effects of Amphetamines

Disrupted body temperature regulation
Increased blood pressure
Insomnia
Increased diuresis and body-water losses
Depression
Increased heart irregularity
Increased anxiety
Increased basal metabolic rate, leading to weight loss

NUTRITIONAL AIDS

Nutritional aids are the safest, most effective, and most readily available ergogenic aids. There is a variety of nutritional aids available. As chapter 3 stated, proper nutrition is essential for optimal sports performance. Athletes can get all of their necessary nutrients by eating a varied, balanced diet. While most dietary supplements will not hurt you (some will), they will hurt your wallet.

CARBOHYDRATES

Carbohydrates are the most important fuel for muscular work. Carbohydrates supply increased energy during periods of increased intensity of exercise. Athletes should avoid the intake of simple carbohydrates, such as honey and candy. These types of carbohydrates enter the blood system very rapidly, causing a rise in blood sugar and insulin secretion, which causes the blood sugar level to fall below normal values and reduces rather than enhances performance.

Carbohydrate loading is a method of enhancing the storage of muscle glycogen that increases one's capacity for intense work. A good way of knowing if you have been successful at carbohydrate loading is to weigh yourself during the carbohydrate loading period. Because glycogen binds to water, you will probably gain several pounds during carbohydrate loading. If you want to consume carbohydrates before or during exercise, try some of the commercially available sport drinks. You should try to pick a drink that has a 5 to 6 percent glucose content. Following competition, load up on your carbohydrates again. During an intense athletic event your glycogen stores get depleted, and if you do not replace them soon after, you will continue to be very fatigued for several days following competition. The Fitness Tip on page 144 outlines an effective carbohydrate loading plan.

L-CARNITINE

L-carnitine is a compound essential for the transport of certain fats into the mitochondria for energy production. It is synthesized in the body and is stored in skeletal and cardiac muscle. The theory behind the use of L-carnitine as a supplement is that higher levels of carnitine in the muscle might increase the utilization of fat, and thus spare glycogen levels. To date, the performance-enhancing effects of L-carnitine remain unproven.

AMINO ACID SUPPLEMENTS

Hailed as "natural" anabolic steroids, **amino acid supplements** are supposed to stimulate tissue growth and thus strength development. Some ads claim that taking these supplements will accelerate muscle development, decrease body fat, and stimulate the release of another anabolic stimulator, your natural growth hormone.

Fitness Tip

Carbohydrate Loading Plan	
Day 1	Mixed diet; moderately long exercise bout, but not to exhaustion.
Day 2	Mixed diet; moderate carbohydrate intake; decreased exercise.
Day 3	Mixed diet; moderate carbohydrate intake; continued decrease in exercise.
Day 4	Mixed diet; moderate carbohydrate intake; continued decrease in exercise.
Day 5	High-carbohydrate diet; moderate exercise.
Day 6	High-carbohydrate diet; light exercise or rest.
Day 7	High-carbohydrate diet; light exercise or rest.
Day 8	Competition

In fact, taking amino acid supplements may actually be counterproductive to gaining strength and muscle mass. According to one of the leading experts in the field of protein and amino acid supplementation and exercise performance, Dr. Gail Butterfield, "dietary supplements with individual amino acids may have negative effects and should be taken with caution, if at all." In addition, Dr. Butterfield states, "There is no reliable evidence that increased intakes of individual amino acids will enhance performance or will significantly stimulate the secretion of growth hormone."

Consuming an unbalanced amino acid formula (high in some amino acids and low in others) can cause a negative nitrogen balance and may impair protein metabolism. Large doses of the essential amino acid leucine can inhibit the uptake of isoleucine, another essential amino acid. Substituting amino acid supplements for protein-rich foods can cause deficiencies in essential nutrients such as iron and the B vitamins. And lastly, the human body is better able to absorb dietary proteins in the more complex form that food provides. When a large dose of amino acids reaches the intestines (the site of absorption) water is drawn into the intestines, which can cause irritation, cramping, and diarrhea.

Taking amino acid supplements can be quite costly compared to eating high-protein foods (Table 14-1). The amount of protein or amino acid found in the special powders or pills is far less than that obtained from foods. You decide, what do you think is the best source of dietary protein, food or supplements?

TABLE 14-1

Amino Acids: Food Versus Supplements

Food or Protein Supplement	Amount	Arginina (mg)	Tryptophan (mg)	Amount Needed for 25 g Protein	Approx. Cost $
Chicken breast	4 oz. (raw)	2100	400	3 oz. (cooked)	0.30
Eggs	2	780	200	4	0.35
Skim milk	1 c	300	120	3 c	0.55
Amino fuel	1 svg	20	75	7 wafers	1.45
Coach's formula	1 svg	410	170	5 T	1.10
Dynamic muscle	1 svg	680	240	4 T	0.70

Source: *Nancy Clark's Sports Nutrition Guidebook.* Leisure Press, 1996.

CHROMIUM

Chromium supplements work by increasing the sensitivity of insulin receptors. Although insulin is an important anabolic hormone, chromium supplementation has not been definitively proven to aid in strength development or improve athletic performance.

VITAMINS AND MINERALS

Most athletes consume more than enough vitamins with a normal diet of 2,000 to 2,500 calories. Unless your diet is significantly deficient in the basic food groups, or you are on a starvation diet, vitamin and mineral supplements are not necessary. Furthermore, there is little scientific evidence to demonstrate any effect on performance from taking vitamin or mineral supplements. The minimum daily requirements are easily met through a varied, balanced diet.

> Taking vitamin or mineral supplements above the minimum daily requirement does not increase physical performance.

WATER AND ELECTROLYTES

Drinking plenty of fluids is essential for all athletes. Fluids transport nutrients to and from the working muscles, help dissipate heat, and eliminate waste products. Unfortunately, few athletes understand the importance of adequate hydration. It is important for athletes to drink plenty of fluids before, during, and after an athletic event. Drinking a fluid containing a small amount of electrolytes and carbohydrates can enhance performance and improve recovery time.

SUMMARY

- You do not need to take drugs to be a successful athlete. Taking legal or illegal drugs to enhance your performance will only hurt you in the long run. Taking drugs also hurts other people in your life besides yourself, like your friends and your family.
- An ergogenic aid is any substance, process, or procedure that may, or is perceived to, enhance performance.
- There really is no good reason to take any kind of drug.
- Anabolic steroids are natural hormones that make it easier for some cells to form additional protein. Steroid hormones increase the rate at which muscle gains and tissue repair occur.
- Synthetic steroids are very dangerous because of the lack of regulation in their production and distribution.
- Young athletes who take steroids before reaching puberty risk causing a premature fusion of the growth plate in the bones, leading to stunted growth.
- There is little substantial scientific evidence to suggest that growth hormones, amphetamines, vitamins, or amino acid supplements increase strength, power, or athletic performance.
- Carbohydrates are the most important fuel for muscular work.
- Drinking plenty of fluids is essential for all athletes, because fluids transport nutrients to and from the working muscles, help dissipate heat, and eliminate waste products.

▶ **Amino Acid Supplements   p. 143**
Nutritional supplements that are thought to stimulate tissue growth and thus strength development.

▶ **Amphetamines   p. 142**
Synthetic drugs that produce stimulation of the central nervous system.

▶ **Anabolic Steroids   p. 139**
Natural hormones formed in the testes and the adrenal glands. Natural and synthetic steroids increase the rate at which muscle gains and tissue repair occur.

▶ **Carbohydrate Loading   p. 143**
A method of enhancing the storage of muscle glycogen that increases one's capacity for intense work.

▶ **Ergogenic Aid   p. 139**
Any substance, process, or procedure that may, or is perceived to, enhance performance.

▶ **Growth Hormone   p. 142**
A protein secreted by the pituitary gland that helps support growth and the development of body tissues.

Appendix

Twelve-Week Complete Body Strength Assessment Program

WHAT IS STRENGTH ASSESSMENT?

Strength assessment is the measurement of strength levels prior to, during, and at the conclusion of a strength training program. To be most effective, all of the major muscle groups should be included in such an assessment. These major muscle groups include: legs, back, chest, shoulders, arms, and abdominals. There should be at least one strength test for each major muscle group. If you must abbreviate your testing choose two or three multijoint, multimuscle exercises such as the squat and bench press.

WHY IS STRENGTH ASSESSMENT IMPORTANT?

Strength assessment is important for the purpose of charting and tracking progress. Is your program really effective? Are your program goals being met? What percentage of improvement can you expect to see over time with a given program scheme? These questions can be easily answered through program testing.

HOW OFTEN SHOULD I ASSESS MYSELF?

As a general rule, maximum strength tests should not be administered more than once a month. Testing every six weeks to two months is ideal for charting progress. Testing in time periods under these limits could lead to overtraining or injuries. Furthermore, it is unlikely that significant progress will be noticeable in time periods of four weeks or less.

WHAT TYPE OF TEST SHOULD I USE?

A battery of multijoint, major muscle group tests should be selected. Do not choose tests that involve equipment you are unfamiliar with or do not have regular access to. Choose a number of tests that will allow you to get them done in a reasonable amount of time. It may be best to test yourself with a partner, and always make sure proper spotting takes place.

GUIDELINES FOR 1RM TESTING

1. Before starting any training program be sure to have proper clearance from your physician.

2. Prepare for test day by getting plenty of rest. If you are tired or stressed you will not obtain reliable results.
3. Make certain the facility is safe for testing: available first aid equipment, staff personnel trained in first aid and CPR, and available 911 access.
4. Standardize your testing procedures by using the same equipment, exercises, and measurements each time you test.
5. Make sure you and your partner follow proper spotting procedure. Do not be afraid to ask around the gym for extra help when needed.
6. Before testing, follow adequate warm-up procedures. Perform several sets leading up to approximately 85 percent of your 1RM.
7. Use a conservative first attempt. You will usually achieve your true 1RM within three or four attempts. Attempts should proceed from approximately 90 percent of the estimated 1RM to 105 to 110 percent of the 1RM.
8. Rest. Give yourself the opportunity to rest three to five minutes between attempts as needed.
9. If you are testing multiple body areas, proceed from greatest intensity to lesser intensity, larger muscle groups to smaller muscle groups, multijoint to single joint, and from strength testing to muscular endurance testing. It is not recommended to test strength and power (plyometric tests) on the same day or in the same session.

Twelve-Week Strength Assessment Battery for Free Weights

Name:		Body weight:			
Age:		Training level:			
Goals:					
	Week 1		Week 6		Week 12	
Exercise	Pre-Test	Post-Test	Pre-Test	Post-Test	Pre-Test	Post-Test
Squat						
Bent-over row						
Bench press						
Press behind the neck						
Triceps extension						
EZ curl						
Crunch (in 1 minute)						

Note: Test should be completed in the recommended order of exercises listed.

REFERENCES

Bosco, C. 1982. Zur trainingwirkung Neuentwickelter sprung-ubongen auf die explosivkraft. *Leistungsport* 12 (1):36–39.

Dick, F. W. 1984. *Training theory.* London: British Amateur Athletic Board.

Field, R. W. 1987. A comparison of the effects of plyometric training and weight training on power development in athletes. Master's thesis, East Stroudsburg University.

Mentzer, M. 1993. *Heavy duty.* Mike Mentzer, Venice, CA.

Robergs, R. A., and S. O. Roberts. 1997. *Exercise physiology: Exercise, performance and clinical applications.* St. Louis, MO: Mosby-Year Book, Inc.

Roberts, S. O. 1994. *Strength and weight training for young athletes.* Chicago, IL: Contemporary Books.

Roberts, S. O. 1995. Fitness walking. Indianapolis, IN: Masters Press.

Roberts, S. O. 1996. *Developing strength in children: A comprehensive guide.* Reston, VA: The American Alliance for Health, Physical Education, Recreation and Dance.

SUGGESTED READINGS

Baechle, T. 1994. *Essentials of strength training and conditioning*. Champaign, IL: Human Kinetics.

Gaines & Butler. 1974. *Pumping iron*. New York, NY: Simon & Schuster.

McCallum, J. 1993. *Keys to progress*. Larkspur, CA: Iron Mind Enterprises.

McRobert, S. 1991. *Brawn*. Nicosia, Cyprus: CS Publishing.

Roberts, S. 1994. *Strength and weight training for young athletes*. Chicago, IL: Contemporary Books.

Starr, B. 1978. *Strongest shall survive*. Baltimore, MD: Fitness Products Limited.

Strossen, R. 1989. *Super squats*. Larkspur, CA: Iron Mind Enterprises.

INDEX